W9-BEQ-301

Copyright Notice

First Printing, 2012

ISBN-13: 978-1477421598
ISBN-10: 1477421599

Printed in the United States of America

Table of Contents

Part 1

Introduction To HIIT

Introduction

Thank you for picking up your copy of HIIT - High Intensity Interval Training Explained by me, James Driver.

Who is this book for and what is it intending to achieve?

This book is for those who would like to improve their fitness, lose weight, improve sports performance or simply have fun engaging in the most enjoyable and most beneficial form of aerobic/anaerobic exercise there is.

This book is primarily for those who're new to HIIT, however intermediate and even more advanced participants will also gain a wealth of knowledge from this book.

After reading this book, you'll have the knowledge and confidence to create your own HIIT workouts designed to meet your own goals.

In this book we're going to discuss the following:

- What is HIIT?
- The benefits of HIIT when compared to other methods of exercise such as continuous training.
- The different HIIT protocols.
- The required HIIT intensities, durations and frequencies.
- HIIT modes as well as specific HIIT exercises.
- HIIT best practices.

- Creating your own HIIT workouts geared towards helping you achieve your goals in a time span that I believe no other form of training can beat.
- And more.

So what are my credentials?

I've been a personal trainer for many years as well as a keen advocate and participant of HIIT. I know full well the benefits that HIIT has brought my personal training clients and the benefits that HIIT brings over and above all other forms of training such as continuous training.

I'm intending to keep this book as short as possible; there will be no filler or fluff. As I'm sure you'd agree, the best place to be is not reading a book, but is instead in the park or gym doing some HIIT.

Let's begin the journey.

What Is HIIT?

As the name implies - HIIT, also known as Interval Training (IT) or Sprint Interval Training (SIT) consists of a set number of high intensity exercises, each immediately followed by periods of recovery. The high intensity exercises can range anywhere from between 5 or 10 seconds to 5 or 10 minutes. Likewise the periods of recovery can range in duration too.

HIIT also enables you to mix up the intensities of your high intensity periods as well as your recovery periods.

By keeping everything varied during a workout, your training session remains considerably more interesting when compared to continuous training (CT). During the course of this book, I will be referring to CT many times. I'm sure you're aware of what CT is however, just to clarify CT usually involves exercising at the same intensity for the entire duration of the exercise session; for example, jogging, cycling or swimming at the same speed or intensity for 45 minutes or more.

To attain the maximum benefits from HIIT, with the least time investment, ideally the high intensity exercise periods should be extremely intense, as intense as you can possibly make them. They should fatigue you quickly and you should give them everything you have. However this will only last for a very short duration as exercising at high intensity for extended periods is difficult. This will be due to the rapid build-up of lactic acid as well as a depletion of creatine phosphate (CP) stores, an energy compound in your muscles that powers the body when engaged in extreme high intensity activity. This combination will prevent you from exercising any longer at your current high intensity, at which point a recovery period will be required.

The recovery period should involve light exercise such as walking, gentle jogging or cycling at an easier pace. This will stop blood pooling in your legs, something which happens following exercise without a cool down. The recovery period also assists in the removal of metabolic waste products such as lactic acid. During this time, CP stores will also be replenished, enabling the body to perform high intensity work again, such as sprinting or high intensity cycling. The recovery period is used to prepare the participant for the next high intensity period of exercise which should soon be approaching.

The variables which can be manipulated during a HIIT workout are as follows:

- Duration (time or distance) of high intensity interval.
- Intensity (speed, resistance) of high intensity interval.
- Duration of recovery interval.
- Intensity of recovery interval.
- Number of repetitions of both high intensity interval and recovery interval.
- Mode of workout (running, cycling, rowing etc).

All of this will be discussed in great detail throughout the course of this book.

Why Does HIIT Work So Well? An Evolutionary Look

As living beings, working in intervals is much more natural than working at the same pace constantly. If you think about it, when in our daily lives do we ever work at the same intensity?

From waking up to going to bed, our work rate and heart rates fluctuate all day long. Since our activities change constantly, so does the blood flow around our bodies to supply oxygen and energy to the working muscles when it's in need.

As we were evolving, our bodies learned to use a greater proportion of energy by performing tasks in intervals over performing the exact same task at a steady and constant pace. During the course of any one day; hunting and gathering, climbing, walking and carrying would all involve intermittent bouts of short bursts of high intensity activity. In addition, escaping danger would involve the same kind of short burst, high intensity activity. This was a survival mechanism since we never knew when we would be attacked by predators in such a dangerous world. Our bodies needed to have an explosion of energy ready for us when we were required to run hell for leather from wolves, bears, other animal predators or even from our deadly spear wielding ancestors from rival tribes. I'm sure you can relate to the fact that developing the ability to run long distances at a steady pace would not have enabled our ancestors to catch prey or escape predators. However, developing the ability to sprint short distances at an extremely fast pace certainly would have.

HIIT is what comes naturally. It should therefore be no surprise that we experience superior benefits using HIIT over CT. If you feel the need to relate HIIT to a more modern perspective then simply think about children and what they naturally do in the playground when playing with other children. Do children play at the same pace for an hour at a time? Or do they instead run around for a few seconds or minutes and then stop for a rest? Obviously it's the latter. It's clear that short bursts of high intensity activity is hardwired into our genetics.

As a consequence and to reiterate, we burn more calories naturally by performing any task in intervals over performing the same task at the same rate for a prolonged period of time. This is true as long as the interval reaches a high intensity, such as if you were running away from a spear wielding ancestor. In fact, the higher the intensity the better for your fitness related goals, whatever they are.

Luckily for us, we can apply these principles to accelerating weight loss, improving our cardiovascular system, improving athletic performance and to a range of other exercise related aims.

One of the principal laws of nature as well as human physiology is that we adapt to stress. By maintaining a constant pace of 70 - 75% of our maximal heart rate for a prolonged period of time, as in CT, we simply aren't stressing our bodies anywhere near enough to force it to make the rapid changes we'd be hoping for, especially when considering the huge time investment that many of us put into exercise. However, by reaching a peak of 100% of our maximal heart rate and holding it for as long as we're capable, if only for a few seconds, not being able to push ourselves any more, feeling the lactic acid building up, burning us and hurting us, this will force our bodies to evolve extremely quickly to better be able to cope with these new physiological conditions.

This is evolution. Let's use it to our advantage.

Who Is HIIT For?

The vast majority of people will have no problem with HIIT.

The Trained Individual

For those better trained individuals, HIIT will give you a chance to further improve on your gains and at a much faster pace. HIIT will give you a chance to test your capabilities to the maximum. If you consider yourself cardiovascular trained but have never incorporated any form of HIIT into your training, you should find you'll take to HIIT extremely quickly and will have no problems adapting. The sudden extra shock to your system will force your physiology to make those changes to your fitness at a rapid pace which you've never experienced through CT. I'm hoping and fully expecting you to become a fan and advocate of HIIT.

The Untrained Individual

If you're sedentary or have little exercise experience then it's always suggested you check with a doctor before embarking on an exercise programme to ensure you're fit to take part. This is true for any new exercise programme, not just HIIT.

I want to make extra certain you understand the above point because the whole idea of HIIT is to work at higher intensities when compared to other forms of training, albeit for shorter durations.

While it's true that you can carry out HIIT at comfortable intensities when starting out, the aim should always be to be working as hard as you possibly can; 100% of your maximal heart rate. Ideally you should also be aiming to hold this intensity too, for as long as you're able. The build-up of lactic acid in your muscles, as well as the depletion of CP stores, will be the deciding factor in just how long you'll be able to hold this intensity and it will be different for every participant.

You can and should build up to this level, but it has to be understood that this is where you should be aiming to go, and the sooner the better.

Therefore, if you're an untrained individual, you should start off at the easier end of the difficulty spectrum. You can do this simply by making your high intensity periods slightly less intense and for a shorter duration. You can also increase the length of your recovery periods to something that is manageable. Within a short number of HIIT sessions, you'll be able to increase the intensity and you'll be surprised by just how quickly your fitness improves. I'll provide evidence for this shortly.

For those who are worried about having to reach such high levels of exertion, I will say that there will be times in life when you'll be required to use bursts of high intensity and all-out effort. Imagine the next time you're rushing to catch a train or plane, carrying two heavy bags of luggage. Perhaps you have a family emergency you need to attend to and you need to be home as quickly as possible. You'll not think twice about the level of exertion needed to get home under such circumstances. How about when somebody snatches your bag, wallet or cell phone? Wouldn't it be preferential that you had training for when the time arrived?

Of course you'll leave plenty of fuel in the tank when just starting out and will ease yourself gradually into the all-out efforts of HIIT over a few weeks. Nobody is asking anybody to become an Olympic athlete overnight. However, when things become easier for you, as they will do very quickly, you should be expected to increase the intensity and not the duration of the exercise. Unlike with CT, intensity is the magic word, and not duration. Quality not quantity!

I have read anecdotal evidence from an elderly gentleman recovering from multiple bypass surgery, who after having been cleared by his doctor, took part in HIIT sessions. The patient made incredible improvements to his cardiovascular system, despite giving up his medication and having complete non-adherence to his prescribed diet. His doctor later told him to carry on doing what he was doing. It appears that HIIT is safe even for people recovering from multiple bypass surgery.

If you're still worried about the risk from such high exertion due to your age or fitness level, I refer you to a study published in the New England Journal of Medicine

[1]. The study showed that the actual risk from any particular bout of vigorous exercise was extremely low; 1 death in every 1.51 million episodes of strenuous activity. Furthermore, the study showed that habitual vigorous exercise, such as HIIT actually lessened the risk from sudden death from the actual exercise itself. One should not be surprised that controlled exercise diminishes the chances of sudden death happening from say, sprinting to catch a train while carrying your luggage.

The Busy Individual

For those people who lead busy lifestyles and are hard pressed for time, HIIT allows you to achieve all the benefits of a longer workout session and indeed more in a far shorter duration. Due to many years of fitness advice and propaganda, people believe wrongly that to lose weight and to build a healthier body and heart requires a great deal of continuous training, which of course requires a great deal of time. Studies show that the number 1 reason for non-compliance to exercise programmes is a lack of time. With HIIT, this can no longer be used as an excuse.

If you're the type of individual who spends much time away on business trips, staying in hotels or on vacation then rest assured that with HIIT, there's little need for any equipment and in some instances, there's no need for a great deal of space either.

As I'll demonstrate through the use of studies in this book; HIIT is also suitable for everybody from children to elderly cardiac patients, from the highly trained to the sedentary and overweight.

Part 2

HIIT Versus Continuous Training

HIIT Versus Continuous Training

I thought the best way to begin this book would be to motivate you by highlighting the large gap in potential achievements when comparing HIIT to CT, taking into account a range of common exercise aims. As you'll see, HIIT is superior to CT in every way.

We'll now compare the two training methods in the following areas:

- Exercise Enjoyment
- Weight Loss
- Exercise Duration
- Improved Fat Burning Capacity
- Anaerobic Threshold
- Beta-Endorphin Levels
- Maximal Oxygen Uptake / VO2 Max
- Athletic Performance

Exercise Enjoyment

When most people begin an exercise regime, they assume that CT is the only form of aerobic exercise there is, even though there are many things you can do with CT; treadmills, cycling, rowing, skipping, stair climbing, elliptical trainers etc. Due to the usual fitness advice that new exercisers receive, they envisage many hours toiling away while staring at a blank wall.

For most people, CT soon gets boring. Exercising at the same, or very similar levels for 45+ minutes can be rather monotonous for the vast majority of people. Surveys repeatedly show that boredom with exercise is one of the main reasons people give up. I'm sure you can relate to this. What can be more boring than sitting on a stationery exercise bike (or insert machine here) for 45 minutes, peddling away at the same speed and intensity for the entire duration?

With HIIT, because you are constantly changing the pace, it's far more interesting. Informal discussions with clients show that rather than dreading the thought of an exercise session, they actually look forward to the thought of a HIIT session and all it involves. There's something extremely enjoyable about running on full burners for only a few seconds before having a nice gentle stroll, then going full throttle again.

A problem with CT is that the thought of only being ten minutes into your run and having another 30+ minutes remaining and at the same pace can be rather demotivating. However with HIIT, knowing that you're running at an intense pace for only a few more seconds before having a nice easy walk for one or two minutes for example can be pleasing to the mind and can spur you on indefinitely. Working at high intensities is a lot easier if you know you have a rest coming up round the next corner.

This can be backed up by taking a look at a study carried out at Liverpool John Moores University in 2011 [2]. The aim was to compare ratings of perceived enjoyment between one group partaking in HIIT and another in CT.

The first group of 8 men performed 6 high intensity intervals running for 30 seconds at 90% of their maximal heart rate. These intervals were interspersed with 3 minute periods of walking at an easy pace. The second group ran for 50 minutes at a constant pace equivalent to 70% of their maximal heart rate. All participants assessed their enjoyment by using the Physical Activity Enjoyment Scale. This scale consists of 18 questions where subjects rate their enjoyment on a scale of 1 – 7. The higher the scores – the greater the enjoyment.

Ratings of perceived enjoyment in the HIIT group were rated at 88 points whereas the CT group rated their enjoyment at 61 points. This was despite ratings of perceived exertion actually being marginally higher within the CT group.

But for those reading this book who regularly participate in HIIT and for those who are about to find out for the first time – The fact that HIIT is more enjoyable than continuous training should come as no surprise.

Weight Loss

Studies have indeed shown that when it comes to weight loss, HIIT is far superior to CT.

In 2011 at the University of Western Ontario [3], 20 men and women were assigned randomly to a HIIT group or a CT group. In the HIIT group, subjects were required to run on a treadmill with 4 to 6 bouts of all out sprints lasting 30 seconds. Each 30 second bout of all out sprinting was separated with recovery periods lasting 4 minutes. The CT group jogged on a treadmill at around 65% of their maximal heart rate for between 30 and 60 minutes. Training sessions for both groups took place 3 times per week for a duration of 6 weeks.

What were the results? After the 6 week study, subjects in the CT group lost a total of 5.8% of their fat mass. This is great news. But what about the HIIT group? Subjects in the HIIT group lost a total of 12.4% of their fat mass.

Feel free to read through the study yourself (all studies used in this book are referenced at the back). The results speak for themselves that HIIT is clearly superior over CT when it comes to fat or weight loss – At least this is true when participating in HIIT sessions 3 times a week over a 6 week period as in the study. But does partaking in high intensity activities provide superior results when they are carried out habitually over a longer period of time? Let's take a look at another study.

In 1990, The American Journal of Clinical Nutrition [4] analysed data taken from the Canada Fitness Survey. In the survey, 1366 men and 1257 women aged between 20 – 49 were analysed for body fatness, fat distribution (waist to hip ratio measurements) and energy expenditure, frequency, intensity and duration of habitual leisure time activities. All data was collected via use of an extensive questionnaire as well as by physiological measurements taken in a clinical setting. In order to determine the effect of exercise intensity on body fatness, subjects from each sex were divided into four sub-groups taking into account the metabolic equivalent of task (METS) value of their leisure time activities; Group A – subjects not reporting activities of 5 METS, group B – between 5 – 7 METS, group C – between 7 – 9 METS, group D – subjects reporting activities of 9 METS or higher.

Before I give you the results, let's take a look at a few examples of METS values; Sleeping scores a METS value of 0.9, walking at 3 mph (4.8 km/h) gives a value of 3.3 METS, whereas for HIIT purposes, sprinting or rope jumping would give a METS value of 10. Every single activity in existence has been given a METS value, which effectively grades the physical intensity of the given activity. If you're curious about how intense your job or favourite hobbies are considered then simply carry out a web search for the *Compendium of Physical Activities*.

The results of the study showed that group D had the lowest waist to hip ratio, lowest waist circumferences and lowest body fat percentages over all other groups and in both sexes. This held true despite group D actually expending a similar amount of total energy during activities as did group A but *much less* than participants in groups B and C.

Let's clarify here that in the study, participants in group D expended similar amounts of energy *during* activities as did group A (but less than groups B and C), yet their body compositions were completely different.

Clearly there are other factors coming into play here and of course we'll be discussing them shortly.

So why is HIIT so superior for weight loss over CT? Well there are two main mechanisms for this.

It has long been known in physiology that when you increase the intensity of the exercise; you actually increase the rate of carbohydrate metabolism and therefore decrease the rate of fat metabolism.

You're probably thinking that if you want to lose weight, or more specifically you would like to lose fat then this would run counter to achieving your aims.

However, when you increase the exercise intensity, you also increase the total caloric expenditure, in fact the total caloric expenditure increases exponentially.

So if you burn a greater percentage of fat calories from lower intensity exercise, the total number of fat calories actually burned off is far lower due to the lower total amount of calories actually used in the activity. Whereas if you increase the intensity; you'll burn off a lower percentage of fat calories but from a far higher total caloric expenditure. If you think about the logic behind this; a lower percentage of a greater number is far more than a higher percentage of a much lower number.

Unfortunately there remains many health care professionals that don't quite understand this logic and so their patients and clients never experience the benefits that come from higher intensity activities. It is understandable to assume that by engaging in lower intensity exercise, patients would be oxidising a higher proportion of fat to carbohydrate than by engaging in higher intensity activities and so this approach would appear superior for weight loss. By considering the energy spent during exercise, this hypothesis seems to be justified on some levels. However, as we are beginning to learn, this simply is not true. Clearly there are other factors working here, such as what happens post exercise. It's these post exercise mechanisms that are too often overlooked, even by health care professionals and many personal trainers, especially when it comes to cardiovascular training.

The other mechanism is *excess post exercise oxygen consumption* (EPOC). Please read the section entitled *Improved Fat Burning Capacity* below as we'll be discussing EPOC in great detail there.

And another thing - Take another look at the study [3] above. There's one thing in that study that the sharp eyed reader will have noticed. This brings us to our next sub-heading.

Exercise Duration

Look again at the duration of exercise in the two subject groups above. What do you spot?

When reading this study, you'd think there was some kind of a mistake. In fact for the study to have been fair, both groups really should have had similar exercise durations but this wasn't the case.

In the study, the CT group exercised for an average of 45 minutes per session. Compare and contrast that to the HIIT group that exercised only for an average time of 22.5 minutes per session. You read that correctly; the HIIT group exercised for precisely half the time of the CT group. Yet by the end of the study and the subjects all had their body fat percentages taken again, the HIIT group had lost more than double the fat that the CT group had lost; 5.8% in the CT group and 12.4% in the HIIT group.

The study shows without doubt that you can lose more than twice the amount of body fat by performing half the amount of exercise with HIIT over CT.

In practical terms, this means you can shorten your HIIT session considerably and still attain superior benefits over and above a much longer and less interesting CT session.

Are you beginning to see the benefits of HIIT now? I urge you to read the study [3] for yourself.

In fact, what is the number one reason why most people claim not to take part in any fitness activities? It's not out of laziness or lack of money, but instead lack of time is cited. By making proper use of HIIT, you can attain superior benefits over CT with only a fraction of the time being invested.

As I mention other studies in this book, please make note of the exercise durations of the two study groups involved as this will push home the above point even further.

So we've established that your HIIT sessions really don't need to be that long in order to achieve incredible and even superior benefits over CT. But how much time during the actual week must you put in? How many individual exercise sessions should you take part in to see these benefits?

Well in the study above, a 12.4% reduction in fat mass was achieved in just three individual sessions per week (for 6 weeks). I'm sure I don't need to tell you just how incredible this is.

However, I can refer you to one study [5] that tested the results of only a single bout of HIIT per week on cardiovascular mortality; cardiovascular disease being the single largest cause of death throughout the entire world.

This study was truly huge, monitoring 56,000 men and women over a 16 year period.

The results were that for cardiovascular disease prevention, a single weekly HIIT session significantly reduced the risk of death in both men and women. Interestingly, they discovered that increasing either the duration of a single HIIT session or the frequency of weekly HIIT sessions had no additional benefits when it came to prevention of death from cardiovascular disease.

This study goes to show that if your goals are not weight loss, but more fitness maintenance and disease prevention, all you really need is a single 22.5 minute session per week in order to achieve this. In reality, who can now cite lack of time as an excuse for not exercising?

Improved Fat Burning Capacity

It is known that the more you exercise the greater fat burning potential your body creates for itself. What I mean by this is that the more you exercise, over time your body becomes more efficient at burning fat no matter if you're out and about engaging in your daily business or even when you're sat on the couch watching a movie.

Why is this? There are several mechanisms within the body that makes this the case.

Increase in Mitochondria

The first of those mechanisms is the increase in the number of and the size of the existing mitochondria within the muscle cells.

Mitochondria are known as the cells "power houses" as this is where glycogen is oxidised and energy is created. When we exercise, over time the increase in mitochondria and their efficiency enhances the body's ability to burn fat for us.

So how does this increased capacity compare between HIIT and CT? Let's have a look at another study [6].

At the University of Guelph, Ontario in 2008 the study was intended to observe HIIT and its ability to improve the body's fat and carbohydrate metabolic capacities in untrained individuals.

The subjects took part in 10 x 4 minute bouts of high intensity cycling separated by 2 minute recovery periods. Exercise sessions took place 3 days a week for a duration of 6 weeks.

At the end of the study, a resting muscle biopsy was taken and there were found to be increases in citrate synthase (26%), a mitochondrial enzyme and 2 different fat transport proteins (14% & 30%). It was found that while cycling at a steady pace of 60% of their maximal heart rate potential, there was a marked increase in fat and carbohydrate oxidation capabilities.

Unfortunately, one limitation of the study was that it did not compare HIIT subjects with CT subjects which would have been interesting to observe.

Just to clarify, the study showed that the marked increase in fat and carbohydrate oxidation capabilities were for CT workouts *after* the HIIT sessions. This shows that after performing HIIT for a period of time and then returning to CT, your body has become more efficient at burning fat.

In another study at the same university in 2006 [7] 8 women took part in 10 x 4 bouts of high intensity cycling with two minute recovery periods.

The subjects took part in 7 exercise sessions over a two week period.

At the end of the study, fat oxidation capabilities had increased by 36%.

Yet again unfortunately, there was no CT group to compare results to. You'd hope they would have learned their lessons at this university but the good thing that came out of the study was that you can see incredible increases in fat burning potential after only 7 exercise sessions. This is the power of HIIT.

However I will now bring your attention to another study [8] that took place at McMaster University in Ontario in 2006. I'm assuming there must be some kind of rivalry between the Ontario institutions to become the authority in HIIT research.

16 men were randomly assigned to either a HIIT group or a CT group. Each group performed 6 training sessions over 14 days on a bike. The HIIT group took part in 4 – 6 x 30 second all out bouts of exercise with 4 minute recovery periods between. The CT group took part in 90 – 120 minute bouts at around 65% of their maximal heart rate.

The muscle biopsy samples taken before and after the study showed that there were similar increases in fat and carbohydrate oxidative capacity in both groups.

But yet again - what stands out from the study above?

Take another look at the overall exercise durations for both groups because the differences here are massive indeed. The HIIT groups exercise sessions lasted for an average of 22.5 minutes compared to the CT group which lasted for 105 minutes. Over the duration of the study this works out at 2 hours 15 minutes (HIIT) and 10 hours 30 minutes (CT).

There you have it. With only a fraction of the exercise duration, HIIT is comparable to CT when it comes to increasing muscle fat and carbohydrate oxidative capacity.

Excess Post Exercise Oxygen Consumption (EPOC)

The second mechanism I referred to is termed oxygen debt or excess post exercise oxygen consumption (EPOC). If you read a lot on the subject of health and fitness then you may commonly hear EPOC described as the *after burn effect*.

When you exercise on full burners as you would with a HIIT session, the aerobic system alone cannot possibly supply you with enough energy to fuel the activity. Although it will do its best and give you all it has, the anaerobic system will have no choice but to come into play to provide extra energy assistance. This point typically comes in at between 65 – 85% of your maximal heart rate, as we'll discuss in the next section.

I will explain the principle of EPOC with the help of an example. Imagine you were going for a swim from one side of a lake to the other. You knew it would take an hour to complete this swim so naturally, you decide to pace yourself. Even if it was your goal to reach the other side of the lake in as fast a time as possible, you would still pace yourself so you wouldn't run out of energy too soon. But what if a shark suddenly appeared and started to swim towards you? Luckily you see a large rock directly in front, about a minutes swim away; so you turn on the full throttle and give it everything you have to reach the rock in order to save your life.

Now, would you say you would be breathing harder after reaching the rock or after reaching the other side of the lake? Of course the answer is that you'd be breathing harder after reaching the rock. This is because turning on full burners has placed immediate and great stress on your aerobic metabolism; this is partly why you're breathing so hard.

A very basic evolutionary and physiological principle is that your body adapts to stress. So if you escape from sharks on a regular basis, or better yet, mimic the shark part in a more controlled environment such as a swimming pool then your body is going to change for the better.

Another reason why you are now breathing harder after reaching the rock than when you reach the end of the lake is because you are now requiring additional oxygen to replenish significant energy stores that were used in haste via non-oxidative metabolic pathways (see Energy Systems below) in order to save you from the shark.

Now this part is very important; you will now need to deal with the incredibly large amounts of lactic acid that have built up in your muscles during the swim as a result of turning on the full throttle. The build-up of lactic acid has had nothing to do with the duration of the swim at all, but is there solely due to the high intensity of the swimming, having escaped from the shark.

This elevated level of oxygen consumption, which will last for several hours, will continue to have a training effect on the body. This is what is meant by the term EPOC or the *after burn effect*. You have finished training, yet you are still burning fuel or calories at an elevated rate due to the high intensity of the activity.

Let me reiterate that there is no EPOC from CT because the activity is just not intensive enough. EPOC is only gained after high intensity activity. How long will EPOC last for? That all depends on exactly how intense the activity was. The more intense the activity – The greater the EPOC. Naturally, the effect of EPOC is at its maximum during the first few hours post exercise when the body has the greatest need to recover. The effect of EPOC then gradually diminishes over and up to the next 48 hours – The harder the intensity of the prior activity, the longer EPOC lasts.

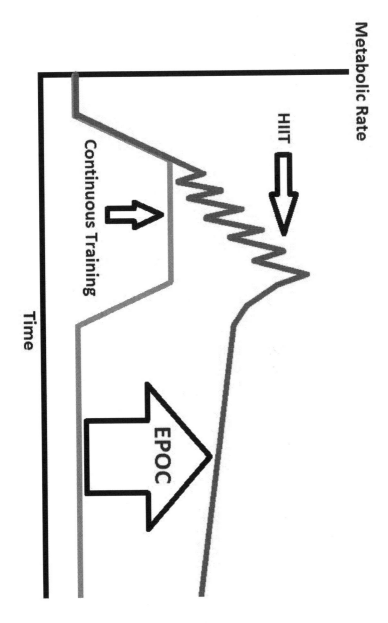

Are you now imagining the physiological benefits that are possible by engaging in regular and sustained HIIT? The potential is massive.

So why else are there such incredible differences in improvements between HIIT and CT?

Well this has to do with the body's energy systems. There are three energy systems in total; the ATP system, the glycogen or lactic acid system, finally there is the aerobic system.

Energy Systems

Each system uses fat and carbohydrate for fuel in different frequencies. Each system is used in different proportions depending on the exercise intensity. They are working all the time in the background and slide in and out of action depending on what we're doing.

The ATP system is used for high intensity work such as sprinting and lasts usually for 10 seconds or less before becoming depleted. The term ATP refers to *adenosine triphosphate* which is in rare supply in the body, but don't worry, once it runs out the body can quickly make it again, luckily for those who do HIIT regularly.

The glycogen/lactic acid system lasts for a bit longer, usually for between 30 seconds to up to 3 minutes and beyond depending on your fitness. Glycogen is the body's supply of fuel which it uses for everything; it tends to be made available to order.

The aerobic system is the system we use the vast majority of the time; when we're eating, sleeping, watching TV or performing very light to moderate exercise.

When we perform CT for long periods, we are only in effect using the one energy system; the aerobic system. It's only when we cross the 65 – 85+% of our maximal heart rate threshold (depending on how fit you are) does the glycogen system come into play. This is where we are in effect utilizing energy on two levels. This is the spot we must aim to hit (or even higher), albeit for only a short duration when partaking in HIIT. In fact in HIIT we should aim to go for 100% of our maximal heart rate in order to train our ATP system also. This way we're utilizing energy on three levels, not two and not one.

Unlike CT, HIIT gives a workout to all three energy systems and not just the aerobic system. This gives us an all-round better workout and has many physical benefits for us that a less interesting CT session can't touch.

By participating in HIIT, you receive a large increase in post exercise fat burning over and above what CT can do. You should think of this as free training time because you have ended your workout session, but your body is still burning fat at an elevated rate.

To clarify this point a little more, I'll reference a study [9] that showed that 24 hours after a HIIT session, HIIT subjects were still burning calories at an elevated rate, whereas the CT subjects were not. Over the 24 hour period that followed HIIT sessions, this equated to an extra 100 calories burned over the CT group. This is quite significant and why HIIT participants can burn more energy and lose more fat by carrying out a lot less work than CT participants.

To really hammer home the fact that you continue to burn fat at an extremely elevated rate following HIIT workouts, I will reference another study [10] that took place at Laval University in Quebec in 1994. The study was designed to discover the outcome of CT and HIIT on body fatness and muscle metabolism.

32 men and women were assigned randomly to a CT group or a HIIT group. The CT group took part in a 20 week programme whereas the HIIT group took part in a 15 week programme. By the end of the protocol, the mean estimated energy cost of the CT group was 120.4 MJ and the mean estimated energy cost of the HIIT group was 57.9 MJ.

Now consider that these figures represent the energy cost from the exercise activities only and not with the inclusion of EPOC. Consider also that the CT group's exercise programme lasted for a full 5 weeks longer than that of the HIIT group. This isn't how I would have designed the study, but let's run with this.

At the end of the study, body fat skin fold measurements were taken and the HIIT group were found to have undergone a reduction in body fat a full nine times greater than that of the CT group.

Read that again.

Nine times greater!

All this despite the amount of energy actually used during the exercise activities were more than two times greater in the CT group over the HIIT group.

Clearly the only way this can be explained is that there are energy sapping physiological changes taking place only following exercise that produces high quantities of lactic acid (HIIT). It further goes to prove that it's not about the duration of exercise, but the intensity.

I'm sure you've heard of the old saying "no pain – no gain" which was coined by Benjamin Franklin.

It appears it really is the truth.

Anaerobic Threshold

What does the *anaerobic threshold* refer to? It refers to that moment when you cross over from the aerobic system to the glycogen/lactic acid system. When exercising at any given intensity, lactic acid builds up in the bloodstream. The higher the intensity, the faster it builds up. When exercise intensity increases to an extent where the production of lactic acid is in excess of its rate of removal/metabolism in the blood then it inevitably builds up to a more noticeable concentration where we begin to feel pain. This is termed the anaerobic threshold.

In real terms, when exercising it's that moment when the painful, performance inhibiting build-up of lactic acid can be felt in the muscles.

Typically, in untrained individuals, the anaerobic threshold will arrive at around 65% of the maximal heart rate. The fitter the individual is, the higher the anaerobic threshold.

Therefore if we only carry out CT work then we will seldom cross over the anaerobic threshold.

What problems does this bring? Well it means you'll not be training your other energy systems.

When we cross over the anaerobic threshold repeatedly such as during HIIT, we're in fact regularly training the anaerobic energy systems (glycogen/lactic acid system and the ATP system). So what effect will this have on us?

Because we are creating more lactic acid within our muscles, our bodies will have to adapt to this. Over a short space of time our anaerobic threshold will be pushed back. So instead of feeling that painful lactic acid build up at 65% of your maximal heart rate, you'll now be feeling it at 70% of your maximum, and then 75%, then 80%. What is happening is that your body is becoming much more efficient at dealing with the painful lactic acid build up, enabling you to work harder and for longer without feeling that burn.

If you push back your anaerobic threshold then by definition, you are increasing your aerobic capacity because the amount of work you can do aerobically has increased in proportion to anaerobic work. In real terms, what effect does this have on your life and functionality?

Well having an increased aerobic capacity can improve your life in many ways, particularly if you were previously deconditioned. No longer will you be exhausted simply by going about your daily routine. No longer will you feel a build-up of lactic acid from taking part in any previously painful physical activity. Can you see how this can improve the quality of life for unfit individuals? You'll be able to go on walks in the countryside, on vacation and play with the kids and not have to break a sweat. If shopping for groceries for example was previously strenuous for you, you should now be able to handle this chore without the feeling of exhaustion you had before.

This is one of the positive training effects of HIIT. We are becoming fitter in ways that CT can't reach. HIIT increases our tolerance to ever more intensive exercise. This is why professional athletes such as Footballers will often train using HIIT since it helps delay the build-up of lactic acid and therefore fatigue. This has obvious benefits for those partaking in sports where there is constant stopping and starting action such as Football, Rugby, Badminton, Tennis, or pretty much the vast majority of sports in existence.

Let's compare the effects of CT and HIIT on anaerobic threshold by taking a look at a study published in the American Journal of Cardiology in 2005 [11].

The study subjects were 14 men who had recently undergone heart bypass surgery. The subjects were split into a CT group and a HIIT group.

The CT group took part in a 10 minute warm up, 30 minutes of training at 65% maximal heart rate followed by a 10 minute cool down. The HIIT group took part in identical warm ups and cool downs. Their training protocol was 2 minutes training at 90% maximal heart rate with 2 minute recovery periods at 40% maximal heart rate. The total exercise duration was 30 minutes, the same as the CT group. The length of the study was 16 weeks and subjects trained two days a week. All subjects rotated training equipment; treadmill, stair climber and a combined leg and arm cycle ergometer to add variation.

Due to the length of the study and to keep everything fair as well as practical, as fitness levels increased, the individual intensity was increased on a daily basis.

Anaerobic threshold was measured by "time to exhaustion" in seconds while working at 90% maximal heart rate. Both groups were measured at the beginning and end of the study.

At the beginning, both groups measured an average time of 100 seconds to exhaustion. At the conclusion of the study, the CT group measured a much improved time of 230 seconds to exhaustion. However, the HIIT group measured a far superior time of 480 seconds to exhaustion.

To conclude; anaerobic threshold was significantly increased in both groups, but to a far greater extent in the HIIT group.

The study showed that HIIT is far superior over CT in giving us a greater tolerance to an aerobic challenge. The study also showed that high intensity training can be safely carried out by an "at risk" group such as those recovering from heart bypass surgery.

By increasing tolerance to hard work to such an extent as this, it should be easy to realise the benefits this would have for the individual concerned. Gone will be the days when thieves could snatch your wallet and expect to make a clean getaway.

Anaerobic Capacity

While *anaerobic threshold* refers to the intensity of work possible before reaching the glycogen/lactic acid system, *anaerobic capacity* refers to the amount of work that can be carried out using both the glycogen/lactic acid and ATP systems. It's the capacity of work that can be carried out between first feeling pain and quitting altogether in a heap on the floor.

I will now demonstrate how compact it's possible to design your workouts while still achieving superior gains by referencing an extremely famous study [12] by a Japanese scientist whose name you may well recognise.

In 1996, Dr Izumi Tabata designed a study with the aim of discovering the effects of CT and HIIT (actually Tabata) on anaerobic capacity.

Using a cycle ergometer, subjects exercised 5 days per week for 6 weeks. The CT group worked for 60 minutes at an intensity of 70% maximal heart rate. The HIIT group worked for 20 seconds at 100% maximal intensity with 10 seconds rest for a total of 8 bouts. The total time for the HIIT workout was – only 4 minutes.

At the end of the study, the CT group were found not to have undergone any significant increases in anaerobic capacity. This is not really surprising considering subjects exercising at a steady state of 70% maximal heart rate would have been unlikely to have passed the anaerobic threshold.

The HIIT group however had experienced gains of 28% in anaerobic capacity. All this from exercise sessions consisting of only 4 minutes.

Now, to many reading this book, you may be thinking - well that's all well and good, but when will I ever need to exercise until I drop? To which I would say – hopefully you'll never have an emergency where you'll need to sprint like your life, or the life of a loved one depended on it. But having an increase in anaerobic capacity should be considered a bonus for any professional or recreational sportsman who regularly delves past the anaerobic threshold.

Just like HIIT itself – Tabata, which is a form of HIIT is becoming increasingly popular the world over. We will revisit Tabata in the *HIIT Protocols* section.

Beta-Endorphin Levels

Beta-endorphin is the "feel good" molecule that is responsible for how we often feel euphoric following an extra strenuous workout.

It's formed in the hypothalamus of the brain as a response to pain. When we feel pain, either emotional or physical, it's soon numbed due to the release of beta-endorphin.

Other functions of beta-endorphin as well as pain relief and giving us the feeling of euphoria is that it's known to slow the growth of cancer cells and it can help us relax too.

Since beta-endorphin is formed when we experience pain stimuli, we know that large amounts are synthesized when we perform strenuous activity such as HIIT. This is in response to the painful feeling of lactic acid that builds up in our muscles; the beta-endorphin tries to dull that pain. Therefore when we only perform CT workouts, beta-endorphin is not created to the same extent.

In fact: "Published studies [13] reveal that incremental graded and short term anaerobic exercise lead to an increase in beta-endorphin levels, the extent correlating with the lactate concentration."

Of course, by "anaerobic" it means a more intense workout such as HIIT. The study showed that a greater amount of beta-endorphin is produced the harder you work out since you'll be creating more lactic acid and the beta-endorphin is created as a response to that.

The study also went on to confirm that beta-endorphin levels do not increase with exercise performed at a steady state, such as with CT unless the CT lasts for longer than one hour. This would explain the "runners high" phenomenon which is often reported by long distance runners.

The whole point of this section is to demonstrate how the "feel good" chemical which affects our moods is more easily created from a HIIT workout over a CT workout and that by training in intervals at high intensity you are setting yourself up for a day in a euphoric state. It has long been known that exercise triggers positive feelings, makes us feel invigorated and is also a great treatment for depression, however the correlation between intensity of the exercise and feelings has not always been known.

Maximal Oxygen Uptake / VO2 Max

It is a person's VO2 max which is often used to derive their overall fitness. According to the American College of Sports Medicine (ACSM), cardio-respiratory fitness is determined by oxygen consumption, technically termed VO2. The "V" stands for Volume, whereas the "O2" obviously means Oxygen. It's measured as a relative rate in millilitres of oxygen per kilogram of bodyweight per minute (ml/kg/min). VO2 max refers to a person's overall capacity to transport and use oxygen during exercise.

As we exercise more and more, this capacity improves as our lungs and heart become more efficient at pumping oxygen rich blood around our bodies to the muscles which in turn become more efficient at using it.

So let's take a look at a couple of studies which compare and contrast HIIT and CT with regards to VO2 max.

In one study [14], 27 heart failure patients with a mean age of 75 were split into HIIT and CT groups. The HIIT group exercised at a rate of 95% of their maximal heart rate. The CT group exercised at 70%. Sessions took place 3 times a week for 12 weeks and VO2 max was measured both before and at the end of the study.

After 12 weeks the HIIT group increased their VO2 max by 46% whereas the CT group increased theirs only by 14%. This is great news for HIIT.

In another study [15], 25 boys with a mean age of 10 were assigned to either a HIIT group or a CT group. The CT group cycled for 20 minutes per session at 80 − 85% of their maximal heart rate. The HIIT group carried out 30 second sprints on a stationery cycle interspersed by recovery periods for a duration of 20 minutes. VO2 max was measured at the beginning and end of the 8 week study. At the end of the study, both groups showed increases in VO2 max, with the HIIT group being the clear winner.

There you have it. When it comes to improving your overall fitness, as measured by VO2 max, which is as good an indicator of overall fitness that has ever been developed, HIIT is clearly superior to CT.

But what else did you notice about the two studies above?

Well the first study was carried out with heart failure patients, the oldest of whom was 86 years old. In the second study the subjects were young children. Both studies involved strenuous exercise at 95+% of their maximal heart capability.

These studies together go to show that HIIT, despite being highly vigorous is indeed safe and even encouraged for absolutely anybody, no matter what their age or physical fitness.

Have you ever considered being tested for your own VO2 max? There are several ways of going about it. Perhaps the easiest method involves the treadmill or stationery bike at your gym (if you're a member of one). Typically you'll warm up for a few minutes then you will run, walk or cycle with increasing speeds, gradients or resistance until you can no longer perform. Since the aim is to discover the maximum quantity of oxygen your body is capable of taking in, you'll be sent to your limit (be warned) and at this point, the time you lasted until is recorded. This time is then placed into an equation, taking your gender into consideration (as well as age and other factors depending on the equation used).

You will be given a final number which is your VO2 max in millilitres of oxygen per kilogram of bodyweight per minute (ml/kg/min). With this number you can of course compare it to the norms for your age and gender if you choose to. But more importantly, you should keep a note of your score and use it as a benchmark for VO2 max tests in the future. I can assure you that by taking regular HIIT sessions, your VO2 max will increase at a promising rate.

Athletic Performance

Which sports actually involve long periods of continuous activity? There are a few but really not that many; distance running, distance swimming, distance cycling and distance rowing etc.

When you think about it, nearly all sports involve some kind of stopping and starting action. From combat sports like boxing and martial arts, racket sports such as tennis and squash, all the way to team sports such as football, both American and soccer as well as basketball or ice hockey. Also there are track and field sports such as jumping, both long and high, shot putting or any throwing event and naturally there is sprinting too; all these sports as a consequence of short bursts of high intensity action will involve the rapid build-up of lactic acid.

Therefore dealing with this painful performance crippling lactic acid is of paramount importance to all athletes or even to the recreational sportsman. If you are unable to deal with high lactate concentrations then you will be at a major disadvantage when compared to any opposition who *is* HIIT trained. And not just your opposition either – But you will also be up against anybody vying for that same position as you on the sports team, for example, your teammates.

As with anything in life, if you want to get good at something then you need to practice it. So if in your sport there is a need to deal with high concentrations of lactic acid, then in order for your body to get good at removing it, you're first going to need to produce a lot of it. Your body will soon find the best way of dealing with the lactic acid and you will adapt as a consequence. By now you should be well aware that HIIT is the single most effective method of creating this lactic acid build-up.

By now you may not be surprised to know that the improved ability to deal with lactic acid build-ups can come extremely quickly by partaking in HIIT. One study [16] has shown that only six sessions of HIIT over a two week period can significantly reduce the build-up of lactic acid in the legs following high intensity cycling.

Having a superior ability to deal with lactic acid build-ups in your body will give you a significant advantage over your opponents and yes, dare I say it, even over your own team mates providing you're involved in a team sport and your selection is far from guaranteed.

But let's not pretend that HIIT is an alien concept to endurance athletes. You may be surprised to realise that HIIT can in fact encompass as much as 50 – 75% of the total training workload of elite endurance athletes. After all, what endurance athlete does not want to be better able to deal with lactic acid build-ups? As already established, what is the superior training method for creating an abundance of lactic acid? Of course, we know it's HIIT. Do you imagine that elite distance cyclists such as Bradley Wiggins or distance runners such as Mo Farah simply ride or run all day long to achieve such high levels of aerobic fitness? Not at all!

Olympic gold medallist and Tour de France winner, Bradley Wiggins: "I do the same warm up every time I ride, and have done for ten years. I do 7 minutes working at an easy 60% of my maximum heart rate with a heart rate monitor, then 8 minutes working at 85%. Then I spend the next 5 minutes doing a series of intense 6 – 10 second sprints, interspersed at 95% with easy 20-second recoveries. It's a routine anyone can follow and benefit from." And that's just his warm up.

While not strictly an *endurance* athlete, let's also consider double Olympic gold medallist in the 1500m and double silver medallist in the 800m – Sebastian Coe. While Coe did indeed regularly train at long distances, he was in fact known for utilising a type of interval training back in the 1970's. Coe regularly set training sessions where he would carry out 200m sprints with 30 seconds of recovery between each run. As well as that, he would frequently carry out as many as 30 bouts of 100m sprints on a hill. After each sprint to the top – He would simply walk to the bottom and repeat.

Of course, the optimum ratio of CT to HIIT for endurance athletes is a matter of constant debate and is far from settled however, what is clear is that all successful endurance athletes will include a significant amount of HIIT in their training regime. It would make perfect sense too; if they want to enjoy all the benefits that HIIT brings and in a time frame that CT can't match or even come close to.

Admittedly, many of these elite endurance athletes will work at the lower end of the high intensity spectrum and for longer periods, which is not what I am advocating for in this book. I would say, as I've provided evidence for already that these elite endurance athletes would benefit greatly from an increase in intensity and a decrease in duration. But this debate will no doubt continue.

What evidence do I have for making these claims? Let's consider VO2 max again and its importance for endurance athletes. Although VO2 max is associated with endurance work and not short bouts of high intensity, we have already established that high intensity exercise does better improve VO2 max over and above more specific endurance exercise – Quite a paradox when you think about it. It's perfectly reasonable to assume that an athlete with a VO2 max of 70 (ml/kg/min) will be able to perform at a higher level and for a longer period than an athlete with a VO2 max of 60 (ml/kg/min).

In a study involving competitive cyclists examining the effects of five different interval training protocols on 40km time trials (17), it was found that the training protocol with both the shortest and most intense interval periods produced the greatest improvements in time along in equal measure with the longest and least intense interval training protocol. These interesting results could most likely be put down to the longer and less intense protocol being the most specific to the actual time trial they were training for. With the shortest and most intense protocol out of the five groups ending in similar results, the author of the study expressed his surprise and made the declaration that the improvements in times were most likely down to an increase in VO2 max.

Summary

If you're new to fitness, HIIT or even if you're a more advanced participant, you're probably wondering just how HIIT is superior to CT in almost every single way.

It has to do with how we adapt and evolve. For the body to make any physiological changes, you have to place it under stress. Without placing the body under the need to change, it's not going to change.

By performing CT we just aren't placing the body under enough stress for it to make any meaningful changes – At least not in an ideal timeframe. CT involves maintaining a steady rhythm that we are comfortable or only slightly uncomfortable with.

When we perform HIIT we are challenging our bodies. We are placing it under severe stress, far more stress than a CT workout would achieve, albeit for a short period of time. Evidently that's all it takes.

When we run, cycle, row, skip or swim at 100% of our maximal heart rate, we accumulate lactic acid extremely quickly, we feel that burn, we deplete our ATP stores and we use all three energy systems. We therefore force our bodies to make bigger, better and faster changes.

In the interest of fairness, it's important I list the benefits of CT too. In no way am I putting down continuous training. It is after all a fantastic method of burning calories, although not as good as HIIT, as has already been demonstrated. CT is obviously better than being sedentary. In addition, in many cases and depending on the individual's fitness, it may be advised to begin your fitness lifestyle with a few CT sessions just to ease yourself into it. Even existing HIIT fanatics who train regularly would experience benefits from the occasional prolonged CT workout at 70% of their maximal heart rate. A varied workout routine is always advised no matter what the participant's aims may be, and an occasional CT session would provide that same shock or stress to the system that is experienced following those first few HIIT workouts – It is after all, stress that makes us adapt.

Another plus of CT is that it's essential for a number of sports such as distance running and other endurance based sports. Yes, even after everything I've stated above, of course endurance athletes are still going to train in a manner that is specific to their sport.

However, for the vast majority of athletes, coaches and sports scientists it's becoming the emerging belief that high intensity interval training is far superior to continuous training. The only thing that goes against HIIT is the years of fitness industry dogma that advocates for and has always propelled CT.

Let's take the example given by the American College of Sports Medicine (ACSM) which is the largest exercise science organisation in the world. In 1995 they updated their Guidelines for Exercise Testing and Prescription, which replaced the earlier guidelines from 1990. In 1998 these guidelines became the Position Stand for "The Recommended Quantity and Quality of Exercise for Developing and Maintaining Fitness in Healthy Adults." They recommended that healthy individuals, in order to maintain their present physical condition should train at an intensity between 55 – 90% (this intensity lowers for unfit individuals) of their maximal heart rate for a duration of between 20 – 60 minutes, 3 – 5 times per week.

More recently, in 2011 they republished their Position Stand reiterating much the same thing. Except this time they said, "ACSM's overall recommendation is for most adults to engage in at least 150 minutes of moderate-intensity exercise each week." Admittedly and to their credit, they do suggest that this can be achieved either by 30 – 60 minutes of moderate intensity exercise (five days per week) or 20 – 60 minutes of vigorous intensity exercise (three days per week). Although I wouldn't necessarily consider the activity "vigorous" if exercise duration approaches 60 minutes.

However, later they state, "Because of the importance of 'total fitness' and that it is more readily attained with exercise sessions of longer duration and because of the potential hazards and adherence problems associated with high intensity activity, moderate intensity activity of longer duration is recommended for adults not training for athletic competition."

Let's agree that ACSM performs some incredible work (they have over 45,000 members worldwide), they are the global authority in exercise science. But we have already seen from the research above that "total fitness" is *not* "more readily attained with exercise sessions of longer duration."

Consider also that in the same paragraph they appear concerned about *potential hazards* (we will address this in *HIIT Pitfalls*), perhaps understandable in an age of frivolous lawsuits. In addition, consider their very genuine concerns over *adherence problems* (International Health Club Association research shows that 50% of new health club members quit within six months with 90% no longer regularly attending), also stated in the same paragraph, and one begins to sense just why the fitness industry advocates more towards CT than HIIT.

However, the research put forward in this book also demonstrates that HIIT is more enjoyable than CT, not to mention the likely increase in exercise motivation and adherence if people actually knew the other potential benefits they could attain from HIIT. Put together, all this should mitigate those *adherence problems* if only HIIT was given the chance and publicity it deserves.

One book entitled *Exercise and Fitness Knowledge – Fitness Industry Training Student Resource*, quotes ACSM – "The American College of Sports Medicine recommends an aerobic heart rate training zone of 55% to 90% of the maximum heart rate as the exercise intensity necessary to achieve health and fitness training benefits from cardiovascular exercise." And doubtless professional trainers having learned from this resource will concentrate their efforts on CT as the primary method for weight loss, achieving fitness and helping clients achieve their dream bodies – And so the cycle continues.

This dogma, also spearheaded by the powerful mainstream media has labelled CT as "aerobic" or "cardiovascular training." This has led to the widely held assumption that CT and only CT can condition the aerobic system and lead to an improvement in cardiovascular fitness and a loss of weight.

How many times when you were at school can you remember actually having a dedicated HIIT session? My assumption is that unless you had a coach on the "fringe" then the answer will most likely be – Never. Yet incredibly while engaging in any number of sports at school, team or individual, you will of course have been engaging in some form of high intensity interval training. It beggars belief as to why the "link" is seldom made and children from an early age are never taken through their paces with regular HIIT sessions. Things must change - Today more than ever.

Hopefully things will change and HIIT will become the normal and accepted mode for training in the future. Its superior benefits are clear for all to see.

I hope I've proven the superiority of HIIT over CT in the sections above. It is clear that whenever researchers have compared both training types side by side, not only has HIIT normally matched CT in every category, but it usually far surpasses it. Not only that, but it does so in a far shorter timescale to add insult to injury.

Once again, given that "lack of time" is the number one reason cited for inactivity and for not starting or sticking with a training regime, I feel that we really do need to hammer home this point.

Part 3

HIIT Implementation

The Required HIIT Intensity

Throughout the course of this book, I've referred numerous times to 65,70,75% etc of your maximal heart rate. So what exactly do I mean by this with regards to HIIT?

What should already have been made clear is that for HIIT to work to its full potential, you really do have to give it everything you have during the high intensity periods of your HIIT workout. Giving it *everything* should obviously equate to 100% of your maximal heart rate.

So how do you know you're giving it 100%? Or how do you know you're only giving 65% of your maximal heart rate for example during the recovery period?

The first thing you need to do is to calculate your age related maximal heart rate. To do this, use the following equation:

220 – Age

Simple - So if you're 30 years old then your maximum age related heart rate would be 190. This means that if you are exercising at 190 heart beats per minute, you would be exercising at 100% of your maximal heart rate or maximum intensity. This is the spot you need to be hitting for as long as you can manage, which won't be any longer than 10 – 30 seconds.

To calculate 65% of your maximum for example for your recovery period then use the following modified equation:

220 – Age X 0.65

In this instance 65% would equate to 124 beats per minute for a 30 year old.

The 65% is just an example. For the heart rate to return to 65% will require differing amounts of time and/or exertion for different people, depending on fitness levels. You may even want to make this number 70% or 75%, it really is up to you and how you're feeling during your HIIT workout. There are no hard rules here. The main aim is to be re-energized for your next hard bout at 100% intensity. You may feel ready to go again for your next high intensity bout having only returned your heart rate down to 85 or 80%. Likewise, there will be those individuals, especially those beginning their journey with HIIT who would prefer to drop their heart rate down to 65 or 60% before their next high intensity interval.

So now we know what we need to be aiming for, how do we know what our actual heart rate is while exercising? There are two great ways of finding out our heart rate - In fact one of those methods is stupidly simple.

The first method involves purchasing a heart rate monitor. They work extremely well and would be a wonderful investment for those wishing to take HIIT (or any form of cardiovascular training) more seriously. They strap around the chest and the reading is taken on a watch. You can simply take regular looks at your watch to check what intensity you are working at. Any specialist running store will stock quality heart rate monitors and of course you could also purchase one online.

The second method is so simple you wouldn't believe it. It has also been shown in studies to correlate extremely accurately with heart rate monitors.

The Borg scale measures rate of perceived exertion (RPE) on a scale of 1 – 10. All you need to do is simply ask yourself on a scale of 1 – 10 how hard you think you are working. If you consider yourself to be working at an intensity of 10/10 then this will in the vast majority of instances correlate to 100% of your maximal heart rate. Likewise, during the rest period you should aim for a RPE of anywhere between 4 – 8 depending on your skill level and aims for your particular HIIT session. And naturally a RPE of 6/10 would in most cases correlate to 60% of your maximal heart rate.

Heart rate monitors are an ideal way for personal trainers to be able to keep check of just how hard their client is working and also for the die-hard HIIT fan who wants to take things to the next level. However, for the vast majority of people, simply asking yourself how hard you're working and then grading yourself will be sufficient. I know of personal trainers who forgo heart rate monitors completely and use the simple Borg scale. It is after all, less invasive as they don't need to strap a monitor to their client's chests, but most importantly, the Borg scale works perfectly well.

A Consideration

Over the years when I've tried to explain HIIT to laymen, one of the big excuses I've heard from people for not giving it a try is that they can't sprint, cycle or row at fast speeds.

This is irritating because they misunderstand the point of HIIT. The point is not to sprint necessarily, but is instead to work at an intensity of 100% maximal heart rate. Now it just so happens that for many people, an effort akin to sprinting is what will be necessary to achieve this level of exertion. However, for many people, 100% can be achieved by jogging or even fast walking. Speed has nothing to do with it. It's all about heart rate. It's all about intensity. Don't forget also that when cycling, if you crank up the gears, you will be achieving this intensity even though you will not necessarily be going all that fast. Everything really is specific to the individual and activity.

The term "high intensity" is extremely descriptive and will be relative to an individual's fitness levels and capabilities. Jogging at six miles per hour will be an all-out effort for many people but will be an easy stroll for many others. What's important is that you are working at a level that is intensive enough for you, for only a short duration and then you can return to something more manageable during the rest period.

Another Consideration

With HIIT you will begin to see improvements extremely quickly. For example, the speed and duration of exertion which used to be 100% of your maximum will soon become 95 and then 90% of your maximum.

Now it's tempting here to think to yourself, "hmmm, that's a lot easier, I think I'll stretch out the duration of that sprint."

The problem with this is that if you're able to stretch it out, you're obviously no longer working to your maximum potential. It is the fact that HIIT is so intensive which is the major factor in all the incredible changes it can make for you. Intensity is the magic ingredient, not duration as should already have been made very clear. Quality not quantity!

It's great you're making the improvements in fitness and you feel like you can stretch that sprint out for a few more seconds, but instead of making that sprint longer, why not make it harder and faster. In other words, make it more intensive. Speed up or find a hill.

This is the key to successful HIIT.

HIIT Frequency

Apart from all the incredible improvements in health you can attain from HIIT, the other great thing about it is that you can do so without having to put in all that many sessions. You don't even need to put in that much time during each HIIT session either.

So what is the recommendation when it comes to HIIT frequency?

Well, because of the high intensive nature of HIIT and the body's need for recovery, I would recommend you partake no more often than every other day. In fact, every other day is the absolute most you should be doing it.

Like strength training a specific muscle in the gym, you would not work that same muscle on two consecutive days. Why? Because it needs sufficient time to rest and recover. It is exactly the same with HIIT. Your body needs rest.

Yes, three sessions per week is ideal for you if your goal is weight loss or to attain a training effect such as improved fitness and VO2 max.

As I demonstrated with an earlier study [5], if your goal is in fact merely fitness maintenance, then incredibly you can get away with a single HIIT session per week. Just make sure you have a quality session.

So how about the length of your actual HIIT sessions?

As you can see from the studies I've referenced, you can achieve all the wonderful benefits from a maximum of 30 minutes per session. I would therefore recommend that you go with 30 minutes. Certainly as you go above 30 minutes the law of diminishing returns seems to come into play. There is also the issue of the muscle's glycogen stores (see *HIIT Nutrition*), which when working out at high intensities will deplete quickly. Once that happens then performance typically drops and muscle wastage begins – Not what we're trying to achieve with HIIT.

A typical 30 minutes of HIIT should not include your warm up, cool down and stretches; you should consider those separate. We need 30 minutes of hard action here.

The number of intervals you're able to cram into a 30 minute HIIT workout will differ for everybody and will depend on many variables such as what your chosen activity is (running, cycling, rowing etc), whether you're in or outdoors, present state, HIIT experience and present fitness. The HIIT protocol you've opted for (see below) will make the largest difference to the quantity of intervals, both high and recovery, that you fit into a single workout because the HIIT protocol actually dictates this.

What is clear is that as you become more experienced and as your fitness improves, you should aim to decrease the duration of your recovery periods in order to cram one, two, three or even more high intensity intervals into a single workout. There's no need to increase the duration of a single HIIT session in order to squeeze in a few extra intervals. But you can certainly cram more high intensity intervals into a single 30 minute HIIT session.

Remember; quality, not quantity!

HIIT Protocols

I will now make a confession. HIIT is actually one of several protocols or plans which fall under the broader category of *interval training*. In order to clear up any confusion that may exist, I shall explain the subtle differences between them.

Interval Training

Interval training is the broader subject that encompasses all the protocols in this section. Put simply, interval training involves a series of low to high intensity exercises interspersed with periods of rest and recovery. The intervals could possibly be of a more relaxed intensity and not necessarily 100% of the participant's maximum, which is where it's distinguished from HIIT. For example, alternating between slow and fast walking paces would be considered interval training, even though the intensity may be easy for the individual. Once the participant puts maximum effort into the high intensity intervals, then it should be considered HIIT.

HIIT

I'm sure you already know what this is. The predominant principal of HIIT is that for the high intensity periods, work is carried out at 100% maximum intensity. There is more flexibility with regards to the intensity of the rest periods along with the quantity of intervals which are all predetermined by the participant.

With HIIT (as in interval training) the interval durations and intensities are fixed and adhered to rigidly. For example, when running or cycling outside, you can use specific trees or lamp posts as markers for changing speed. You would begin at a manageable intensity and when reaching the first marker then that would be the signal to run faster or crank up the gears and pedal harder. At the next tree then you could either increase the intensity into an all-out 100% effort (if you weren't already) or bring the intensity back down to something easily manageable. If you're using a rowing machine at the gym, then the timer would be used to mark the point where intensity is changed.

The main point is that there needs to be set markers or time periods per interval. For example, if you were running then you could sprint at 100% maximum intensity for 100 meters followed by 200 metres of walking, then you would repeat this process for the pre-specified quantity of intervals. Likewise if you were on the stationery cycle at the gym, you could cycle at 100% maximum intensity for 30 seconds followed by the next 2 minutes cycling at 65% maximum intensity.

Interval training and HIIT are very similar in structure. Except the one difference between the two protocols yields massively different results for the participant. I'm sure you know what that difference is? – Intensity!

Fartlek

Fartlek is Swedish for "speed play" and is unique amongst the interval training protocols. With Fartlek there are no definite requirements to reach the pre-set markers, distances, times or intensities. Where HIIT and interval training are rigid and you stick to predetermined intervals such as by using trees or a set time period as a marker to change intensity, with Fartlek there are no predetermined intervals.

Fartlek stands apart from the rest because of one difference - You simply manage the intensities according to how you feel during the moment.

For example, during the recovery period, if you feel you've recuperated enough to begin the high intensity interval again, so that is the signal to go.

Since there are no markers to end your high intensity period, you simply return to your recovery interval when you feel the desire to rest. Likewise, you'll know when you have your energy back ready for the next high intensity interval.

I have found with clients that Fartlek is ideal for beginners since it's easy to overestimate the difficulty of reaching that far off tree at a high intensity. A full on cycle for 30 seconds may sound easy when planning your workouts, but things may change when mounting the bike. Fartlek gives the flexibility of letting one "off the hook" without feeling bad about it. Conversely and for the same reasons, Fartlek training takes away that marker just up ahead that often gives us that "push" to really hammer ourselves in order to reach that near goal and achieve those incredible results that are possible with HIIT.

Fartlek can still work just as well as HIIT as long as you're tough with yourself, disciplined as well as honest.

By all means, give Fartlek a try. If you're only just embarking on your HIIT journey then it will be perfect for giving you a taste of what's to come. You will however soon find that desire to progress to full on HIIT.

Little / Gibala Method

Given that the most common reason cited for non-compliance to exercise is "lack of time," Doctors Little and Gibala at McMaster University, Canada set out to discover the least amount of time required in order to achieve maximum results through interval training. They were also concerned about the high intensity of HIIT potentially causing difficulties for certain individuals. Therefore they were interested in finding that happy medium that would first - achieve results, second - do so in as time efficient a manner as possible and third – would be manageable for beginners, the elderly, unhealthy and obese individuals [18].

The Little/Gibala protocol goes as follows:

60 seconds high intensity

75 seconds recovery

Repeat for 8 – 12 cycles

Total time: 18 - 27 minutes

Their study involved only six of the above exercise sessions over two weeks and of course, as usual, improvements were found in all recorded measurements (VO2 max, time trial performance, increases in mitochondrial enzymes). It's important to remember and place emphasis on the fact that the above protocol is *not* HIIT, as exercise intensity is not 100% maximal but submaximal.

One other detail that sticks out with this protocol is that the study was carried out using a "fast cycling" method on a stationery cycle and intensities were altered via the changing of resistance. However, as with all protocols in this section – In principle any mode can be used (see *HIIT Modes*) such as running, swimming or rowing.

The Little/Gibala protocol should be considered ideal for those individuals concerned about exercising at full intensity – At least until they are ready for HIIT, this protocol should be considered an ideal starting point.

Tabata

The Tabata method, just like the Little/Gibala method, focuses on getting the most "bang for your buck," or the best possible results from the least time invested. However, where the Little/Gibala method is perhaps best utilised for those individuals just starting out on a training regime or for those people who fall into the "at risk" category, the Tabata method is quite the opposite.

Tabata is advanced - Take a look at the protocol below:

20 seconds high intensity

10 seconds recovery

Repeat for 8 cycles

Total time: 4 minutes

Whereas all other protocols involve longer periods of recovery, Tabata has a work/rest ratio of 2:1. And unlike with the Little/Gibala protocol, with Tabata, you must work at the highest intensity you're physically capable of reaching.

There is a common misconception surrounding Tabata, probably stemming from the many online and video tutorials which focus above all on free body exercises, free weights and kettlebells as a training mode which has led many people to believe Tabata can't or shouldn't be used with traditional cardio modes. But this is incorrect. Just like with all the other protocols in this section, Tabata can be performed using any training mode; running for example as long as the training formula above is maintained. Dr Izumi Tabata himself, in his famous 1996 study [12] actually used cycle ergometers. With cycling, it was fully achievable to obtain the necessary intensity within 20 second periods. It is therefore clear that 20 seconds of 100% maximal intensity activity is enough to achieve the desired training effects, something which by now shouldn't be surprising to readers of this book. As Dr Tabata found out in his study, cycling can be just as effective at achieving this as using free weights or kettlebells.

In the study [12] Dr Tabata found that the 4 minute Tabata routine was comparable to 60 minutes of cycling at 70% maximal heart rate – 5 times per week over 6 weeks when measuring improvements in VO2 max. However, when assessing improvements in anaerobic threshold, the CT cyclists had not experienced any improvements, whereas the Tabata subjects had increases in anaerobic capacity by 28%.

It is a great pity that the Tabata study did not take other measurements into account, such as for losses of body fat in obese subjects. However, considering that the Tabata method is so intense, with such a short recovery period, it is my opinion that Tabata should not be attempted until the participant has sufficient experience in the other protocols first (though primarily HIIT), has built up an improved VO2 max, anaerobic threshold and if overweight or obese, has already commenced losing the excess weight through HIIT. I will reiterate that the difficulty with Tabata, compared to the other protocols is the very short recovery period and this must be taken into consideration by the individual before attempting it. It can be observed from the Tabata study that the subject's average starting point for VO2 max was 48 ml/kg/min which, for a 30 year old male, is considered high.

Taking everything into consideration – Tabata should be seen as undeniable proof of what is potentially achievable through short bursts of high intensity activity, even when the total training session lasts for as short a duration as 4 minutes.

I will say again, that those with weight loss as a goal should refrain from using the Tabata protocol and concentrate on HIIT. I don't say this because overweight individuals cannot be physically fit (and therefore cannot do Tabata) because we know they can be. I say this because research on the effects of Tabata on weight loss at this stage simply does not exist. It would be far better to begin (and stick with) the tried and tested, yet under-utilised HIIT which we already know is perfect for weight loss.

For those individuals who are ready and waiting to test their capabilities with Tabata then good luck to you. As with the other protocols, I recommend a training frequency of every other day.

Summary

As you can see, the primary difference between interval training protocols tends to be the length and intensity as well as number of intervals. The principles are the same for each protocol in that they all involve short bursts of higher intensity activity interspersed with differing lengths of lower intensity activity.

Many of the studies referenced throughout this book have in fact used *interval training* protocols and not *HIIT* at all. Yet you've still witnessed the incredible benefits that have been attained. This should be encouraging to those who still have slight trepidation about the thought of going "full-throttle," since you can still achieve incredible gains by utilising submaximal intensities during your high intensity periods. If you're understandably nervous about your first HIIT workout, then I ask you to begin by using the Fartlek protocol and then progressing to HIIT after a few weeks, or once you feel ready.

Those who are able to undertake full HIIT workouts from the start should also find encouragement in knowing what can possibly be achieved. If you already consider yourself to be "trained" then you should begin immediately with HIIT. You may take more ideas from *Sample HIIT Workouts* later on in this book.

The table below is a summary of all the protocols. Please be aware that with the exception of Little/Gibala and Tabata, the protocols are displayed at the extreme upper and lower limits for time and intensities. This is merely to demonstrate the freedom you have throughout your workouts to tailor them to meet your needs and capabilities and is by no means a license to take things "easy" on yourself by exercising at the lower extremities. There should be no confusion by now that no matter what your physical capabilities may be – You will always reap greater rewards by exercising at the more intense side of the spectrum.

Protocol	Interval Training	HIIT	Fartlek	Little/Gibala	Tabata
High Intensity Interval (Time/Seconds)	< 120	< 60	< 60	60	20
High Intensity Interval (Intensity)	75 - 95%	100%	100%	75 - 95%	100%
Recovery (Time/Seconds)	10 - 240	10 - 240	10 - 240	75 seconds	10 seconds
Recovery (Intensity)	40 - 75%	40 - 75%	40 - 75%	40 - 75%	< 40%
Number of Cycles	4 – 12 >	4 – 12 >	4 – 12 >	8 – 12	8
Total Time (Minutes)	20 - 30	20 - 30	20 - 30	18 - 27	4 minutes

HIIT Modes

Now we're getting more into the practical side of things, we'll now take a look at some of the many possible HIIT modes.

The "best" training method will be completely down to the person involved. In reality, the HIIT training fundamentals can be used on nearly anything you can put 100% effort into; running, cycling, rowing, climbing the stairs or digging a giant hole in the sand.

I encourage everybody reading this book to try a number of different HIIT modes so you can find the modes which are dear to your heart. I recognise that most people, myself included will settle primarily on one single HIIT mode. However, as I'll explain in the summary section, there are extra benefits that can be attained simply by mixing up your training sessions. So please read through the following modes with an open mind and with a view to giving a few of them a fair go, even if you've never tried them before.

The training modes we're going to cover are as follows:

- Walking
- Running
- Cycling
- Rowing
- Skipping
- Stair Climbing

- Stepping
- Swimming
- Boxing
- Kettlebells
- Bodyweight Circuits

Walking

There'll be those who believe that HIIT can't be carried out while walking. To those people I would ask them if they've never walked up a large hill or a mountain with a heavy backpack.

Yes — HIIT can indeed be carried out walking and could in fact be the ideal starting point for the deconditioned individual, senior citizens or for those carrying injuries which are preventing them from running.

It is my belief that walking can be made intense enough for most people to achieve a HIIT training effect. But it should be made clear that when the individual is able to do so, then running should be made the primary focus.

While you'll see below that I don't really agree with HIIT running on a treadmill, with walking, using a treadmill will almost always be a necessity for HIIT. Most people will not be lucky enough to live next to a large hill or a mountain and so simulating these conditions using a treadmill will be essential. In order to achieve the required intensities while walking then for all but the most unconditioned individual - this will require a steep gradient.

Choose a brisk pace that will be a challenge and simply alter the gradients as necessary when entering your high intensity periods. Experimentation with making subsequent training sessions progressively more intense can be achieved by the use of ankle weights, weighted vests or by adding food cans or water bottles to backpacks. Of course, the speed of the treadmill can be altered too.

I must emphasise that if you feel unable to achieve the required high intensities when walking then you must consider some of the other training modes below.

Running

Running is the most popular mode for HIIT. It requires no equipment, no gym pass and unless you have an injury then everybody can do it, no excuses.

With running, you can change your speeds rapidly and easily, which is obviously beneficial for HIIT. It's also easy to set markers for yourself by using trees, lamp posts or any other landmark as signals to change speed (if you're not using the Fartlek protocol).

While yes, you can do HIIT on a treadmill and many may prefer to do so, I personally have found changing the speed on most treadmills to be slow, inconvenient and perhaps a little dangerous. As you may know, there's a time lag when changing settings on many treadmills. If for example you've carried out a 10 – 20 second sprint, then you'll most likely really need to slow down quickly since spending any more time at a full sprint is extremely difficult even for the most trained of sprinters and you really don't want to be at the mercy of the treadmill when it comes to slowing down. In addition - stretching out your arms in order to change speed, while sprinting at full speed is more than a little risky. Of course there are many treadmills that enable you to pre-program your intervals which would eliminate the need to reach forward to change speeds. However, consider the possibility that you overestimate your sprinting capabilities and have to wait an extra 5 – 10 seconds at a high speed before the machine will automatically return to something more manageable. A lot to think about perhaps – But you can see why I much prefer pounding the grass outside instead.

You could get round this whole dilemma by maintaining a moderate speed on the treadmill and by using gradients. You can quite easily reach 100% of your maximal heart rate by maintaining a quick jogging pace or even a fast walk on a steep slope. So if your heart is set on using a treadmill then perhaps using a gradient will be the best compromise. Please make sure that you alter the gradient before the speed otherwise you may end up being surprised at just how hard it is to sprint up a steep gradient.

However, none of this compares to HIIT and sprinting outdoors where you can use real hills for your gradients and not be held back by having to fiddle with buttons when in full sprint mode.

Feel free to disagree with me when it comes to treadmill sprinting. I've had clients who've had no problems. But I wouldn't be doing my job if I didn't at least mention the above.

For those who decide to opt for the great outdoors, and I hope it's the vast majority, there are many things you can do to make your runs more interesting while at the same time adding extra elements of difficulty in order to ensure you're working at that magic 100%. Above all, gradients should be used as often as possible. Find a hill and use it.

There are few more efficient ways of generating the required intensity than hill sprints. Likewise, sprinting through forests or along the beach will be more intense than sprinting on concrete. Packing a backpack with water bottles or food cans can work well too. They tend to roll and jump around the place, so be sure to pack towels or clothes in there to absorb the movement. Ankle weights can work in a similar fashion to a stuffed backpack.

I have one friend who built a customised sled that attached by rope to a weight lifting belt around his waist. He began by pulling along a 10kg weight in the sled. The weights then progressed to 20, 30 then 40kgs. After that he started at 10kg again, but this time he would pull the sled up a hill.

It typically takes him around 20 seconds to complete the run to the top of his hill. By that time he's long finished sprinting and has continued with a jog as fast as he can manage. When he reaches the top, he takes a leisurely walk back to the bottom, sometimes in an arc to give himself more recovery time. When he reaches the bottom, he begins again.

The moral is – You can always make your runs more interesting and more intense.

Cycling

Cycling is also a popular method for HIIT. In fact by cycling outside, you will often be performing interval training to a certain extent without even knowing it. This is because of the natural hills and troughs on any cycle route. Who pedals when going downhill anyway? Instead we tend to enjoy the thrill which would encompass a recovery period to my mind.

You can take this further by using your high intensity intervals to cycle harder or perhaps on a higher gear before changing to an easier gear and taking things easy for your recovery period. You should definitely utilise downhill slopes to recover.

Cycling on a stationary bike in a gym will be far preferential to using a treadmill in my opinion. Changing intensities is simple on a stationary bike; increasing speed on a high setting will be perfect for high intensity intervals, while taking things easy on a low setting will be ideal for recovery periods.

HIIT while cycling is great and you should definitely mix it in if you would normally prefer to run. As you have read; many of the studies referenced in this book have used cycling to achieve high intensities very quickly. Cycling is an ideal mode for the HIIT principles.

You can also take a spinning class. For those who don't know, spinning is an indoor group cycling session and most gyms these days will have classes running. Depending on the instructor involved, you will be taken through your paces at a range of intensities and speeds for around 45 minutes. Be warned; spinning is tough. It is also a lot of fun. You are in charge of setting your own intensities so you will be fully able to cycle at an intensity and speed that will succeed in giving you your lactic acid fix. Check the length of your spinning class. 45 minutes is a long time if you're going to be incorporating a HIIT workout into it. You should consider using the first half of such a session as a "warm up" by using a lower resistance on the bike. Then after the halfway point, crank up that resistance and go for it.

Rowing

In the vast majority of cases, rowing will be performed stationary unless you're lucky enough to live near a lake. Either you love rowing or you hate it and when it comes to HIIT, this is even more so. However, rowing will be another great mode to add to your HIIT inventory so I urge you to at least try it out.

Unlike with cycling, rowing utilises the whole body and so reaching those high intensities can be carried out with ease. Most people will agree that rowing can be incredibly intense, which is what we desire for HIIT.

Most rowing machines have a lever in order to alter stroke resistance. But the best way of increasing intensity is by increasing your stroke rate – effectively rowing faster. Between these two variables, you can make the intensities higher or lower as necessary.

For rowing, due to the position of the back, I must emphasise the use of correct technique and so I would recommend, if you've never used a rower before to speak to an instructor and learn correct form. You'll be pulling back on those handles with full force, straightening the knees at high speed. I must also emphasise that you should never lock out your knees on full extension otherwise this could cause problems down the line. Please have a trained instructor show you correct rowing posture and take you through your first attempt. It too often shocks me, watching people on rowing machines with appalling technique and posture.

However, if you have good fundamentals on this piece of equipment then you'll be able to achieve an incredible HIIT workout.

Skipping

Skipping is so simple. Anybody can skip or else learning can be done in no time at all. It's fun and it's free. Alternating your intensities is also a piece of cake.

I've had debates with other HIIT advocates as to which is the better mode for HIIT; running or skipping. I was on the side of running but it was a tough debate. Skipping certainly has its fans and extreme advocates. In fact, in the interest of changing things up, you should incorporate skipping into your workout every once in a while. Why not?

If you've never skipped before, or struggle with the technique, then keep everything slow until you become used to the mechanics. Keep the weight on your toes, try to be nice and light and make tiny jumps from the floor so you're not wasting any energy. There's no need to jump high when skipping.

I like to make use of a timer that beeps when it's time to change intensity. Others may wish to use an app on their phone. Otherwise you can simply position yourself facing a clock. I will often use the Fartlek protocol as I find it convenient for skipping; simply changing the intensity based on how I feel.

Obviously, to make skipping more intense, all you need to do is speed up. Then slow down to bring your heart rate back down again.

Stair Climbing

This is ideal for those who are pressed for time. Most of us have to climb a large flight of stairs during our working week at the office or even returning home to our apartments. If you can't fit in your HIIT sessions during the week, then sprinting up your flight of stairs will be the best compromise under the circumstances. At least you'll have no excuses for not taking some form of HIIT during the week.

Though using a long flight of stairs as your dedicated HIIT mode will of course work extremely well. There are few things more tiring than running up the stairs which makes this perfect for HIIT. When you get to the top, walk down again and repeat. Do this for a total of twenty minutes. If you would like to make this even more intense, although it's intense enough already, then you can employ the use of weights to hold while running or better yet you can purchase a weighted vest or fill a backpack with food cans or bottles of water.

I strongly hope you'll give stair climbing a try. It is after all about variety and experimenting with different modes to find which you enjoy the most and find more beneficial.

Stepping

Stepping is one of the more advanced methods which will not be ideal for everyone. Why? Because this exercise is extremely intense and vigorous, especially during high intensity periods.

By stepping, I'm not talking about the stepping machines you'll find in the cardio section at the gym, although they too can be used for HIIT. I'm talking about using an actual step.

Upright stepping involves the pattern of: One foot up, two feet up, one foot down, two feet down – Then repeat in rhythmical fashion for the desired training effect.

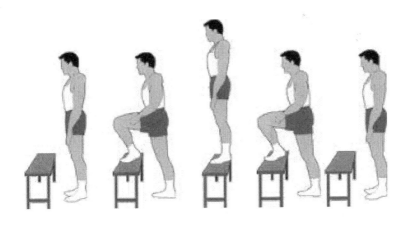

For the high intensity periods you will have a number of options in order to ramp up the heart rate. Most commonly, you can simply speed up the motion of the exercise. Another thing you could do is have a high step for the high intensity intervals and a low step for the recovery periods. You also have the option of using weights or a back pack filled with food cans or bottles of water. Why not use a combination of all these to truly make this an advanced mode of training?

Another advantage of stepping is that it can be carried out literally anywhere; the local park, in the home, hotel room and of course at the gym where setting up stepping boxes of various heights will be easy.

So why is this training mode so advanced when all that's involved is stepping?

Have you ever heard of *delayed onset muscle soreness* (DOMS)? DOMS is what happens following activity with prolonged eccentric movements. The term *eccentric* refers to controlled lowering movements. We perform controlled lowering movements when we put down heavy objects, run downhill or step.

Eccentric exercises cause DOMS, which is effectively a more painful fatigue which manifests following a more prolonged time period post training.

When we carry out a heavy weights session in the gym, training which is predominantly concentric (controlled lifting movements), we will usually feel the fatigue for up to 24 – 48 hours post exercise. However, following a session based largely on eccentric contractions, the fatigue or muscles soreness is not felt until *after* 48 hours and often even later. In the majority of cases, soreness does not dissipate until five days hence.

During stepping, if leading with your left leg, then placing the left foot on the step and then raising yourself up onto it; that movement would consist of a concentric contraction of the left quadriceps. By continuing the motion by leading with the left leg to lower yourself back to the ground then this would constitute an eccentric motion of your right quadriceps as it's this muscle which is controlling the lowering movement. In addition, as the front of the left foot hits the floor, the left calf muscle would be used to eccentrically control the movement of lowering the whole foot flat to the ground. If you don't believe me then try it on a step right now and feel how your toes touch the floor first as your calf muscle controls the lowering of your body.

Therefore, by carrying out a HIIT session involving stepping, these two differing muscles in opposing legs would be feeling the DOMS 48 hours afterwards. It's quite an odd sensation when you have DOMS in this way and one that could result in you walking in circles for a few days.

I took my first dissertation on the effects of post exercise stretching on DOMS and so I know that it's not fully understood why muscle soreness arrives so much later from say stepping than it does with running (unless downhill). But I did discover that (and the existing evidence agreed) post exercise stretching lessened the soreness to a great extent (see below for stretching recommendations). While it did not reduce the amount of time DOMS existed from say 5 days to only 4 – It did reduce the severity of the existing soreness.

If you're an advanced participant, would like to really push yourself and don't mind finding walking a true chore for a while, then upright stepping will be an ideal challenge for you.

Since a good workout balance is always advised, I will also point out that you should alternate leading legs (the front leg carrying out the work) as undoubtedly, the lead leg utilises the muscles in a different way to the trailing leg. Believe me when I say this – You *will* have DOMS following a HIIT session consisting of upright stepping. Instead of having HIIT sessions every other day, as recommended, you'll only be capable of training once every five days. If you don't have much free time then this may well be the right exercise for you, taking everything else into consideration. But in order to add in variety to your workouts, you could always throw in a stepping session once a month or so, at least to try it out.

Swimming

Of course, the HIIT principles still remain intact even when in the water. Swimming has its extreme advocates and flag bearers just like any other HIIT mode.

Swimming carries several advantages that you won't find with the other modes. First – It's low impact and so will be beneficial for those with knee or ankle problems. Second - Swimming will be ideal for those elderly HIIT participants who are perhaps concerned about some of the more high impact modes of training. Third – If you ever find yourself injured then swimming would be the activity that would most likely be recommended due to its low impact nature while the resistance from the water still provides an incredible workout. Indeed when injured, many professional athletes are advised to undertake swimming as part of their rehabilitation.

There are many professional and recreational swimmers who use HIIT protocols in the pool to great effect. While you can of course alter stroke speed in order to increase/lower intensity, emphasis in the pool should always be placed on good form. For that reason, consensus appears to be on altering swim strokes depending on which interval you're presently on. For high intensity intervals then either breaststroke, butterfly or freestyle/front crawl are advised. The latter two strokes in particular are fast paced by nature and therefore naturally vigorous. For recovery periods I suggest using the backstroke as it's slower paced and your face will constantly be out from the water, enabling easier breathing and recovery.

Boxing

I doubt that by now you'll be surprised to learn you can carry out HIIT protocols while boxing. Depending on the kind of day you've had, boxing may even be your preferred choice of workout.

All you need is a heavy bag and some gloves, which by the way I strongly recommend for safety reasons. All gyms will possess these items though purchasing your own pair of gloves may provide you with the extra incentive to give this superb training mode a fair try.

Boxing is ideal for those who may have picked up lower body injuries or who are undergoing rehabilitation anywhere in the lower body.

However, boxing can still be potentially hazardous if correct technique is not utilised. For this reason, I suggest learning proper punching techniques before pounding your fists into a heavy bag at full force. Many health clubs have boxing classes, most commonly Boxercise, but failing that there are hundreds of online videos which demonstrate correct punching techniques. These techniques are often better seen and demonstrated than read about.

There's no need to punch the bag at full force, as simply tapping the bag or punching with medium power is still incredibly intense and carries far less risk of injury. Though feel free to mix in a few hard blows to add variety. And don't forget, you can also add in kicks too. Boxing is a serious workout and so you will feel the burn within seconds.

For recovery periods, it's likely that continuing to punch the bag will be too intense. Instead I suggest jogging on the spot, walking or jogging round the room or light skipping.

Kettlebells

Make no mistake – Kettlebells are back and are becoming extremely popular. Working out with bells can be extremely intense, which of course makes them perfect for us. Most gyms these days have an extensive kettlebell rack.

Like dumbbells, kettlebells come in a range of weights. When performing a HIIT workout using bells for the first time, it's important you don't choose a weight that's too heavy. It's far better to play it safer and go for a lighter weight and then upgrade later, rather than damage your back attempting to swing a weight that's too heavy for you. With bells, we're not going for our 1 rep max. We are instead going for a reasonably sized weight that we can swing with good form, activating a large range of muscle groups in the process.

I guarantee that you'll experience soreness following the first few kettlebell HIIT sessions and naturally this is what you want to try and achieve. But beware of overtraining. If you still feel sore from the last HIIT session then I would suggest refraining from further training until soreness has abated.

There are many exercises you can carry out using kettlebells, but for HIIT purposes it's preferential to use them in a more cardiovascular fashion than simply using them as you would a dumbbell. This means selecting specific exercises that engage as many of the large muscle groups as possible.

Provided below are simple instructions along with a diagram for some of the best kettlebell exercises that fill the HIIT criteria. However, before trying any of these for the first time, I advise further instruction from a qualified gym instructor or at the very least, take a look at a range of explanatory videos online. There are some things that should be seen demonstrated in order to get the feel for correct technique, rather than simply reading about them.

With the majority of exercises in this section – they can be performed with a bell in each hand, one bell in two hands or a single bell in one hand. If you choose the latter then you can alternate hands between intervals. By manipulating these variables as well as the actual weight of the kettlebells themselves, you can constantly make each subsequent training session progressively more intense.

Unlike when doing free weights, with kettlebells, using the momentum is perfectly acceptable. Remember that this is a HIIT workout – The aim is not necessarily to achieve overload in the muscles, but instead to create a heavy build-up of lactic acid.

All movements should be performed in a smooth and fluid fashion. Again, any online training video will show you how they are performed safely and effectively.

With kettlebells perhaps more than with any other training mode, you'll find it convenient to use a timer, HIIT phone app or at the very least a clock to indicate intervals.

I also strongly recommend dynamic stretching (see *Dynamic Stretching*) prior to beginning a HIIT session involving kettlebells.

Clean and Press

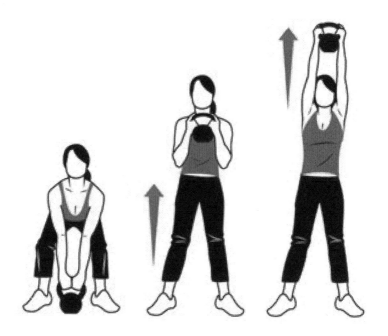

This exercise is carried out in two stages: From the floor to the shoulder and from the shoulder to the overhead position.

Begin in a half squat, taking hold of the bell and with a single clean jerk, pull the weight up to the shoulder. Pause for a beat. Then press the weight above your head. From there, simply allow gravity to assist you in returning the weight back down to the ground. Do not rest the weight on the floor but instead go straight into the next repetition.

Feel free to use the knees to give an extra jerk in order to assist with the raising of the weight during the second stage.

Keep a flat back throughout the entire motion.

Full Swing

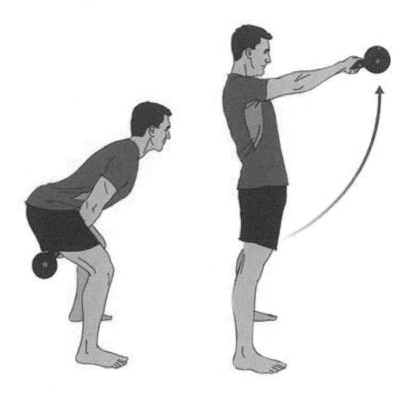

Beginning from a half squat position, swing the bell from between your legs to the arms parallel to the floor position. There is actually the choice of ending the swing motion as the weight is in front of you and your arms are parallel to the floor, or you can continue the motion until it's above your head. Ultimately, the latter will recruit a greater number of muscle fibres to assist with the motion.

The whole manoeuvre is momentum based and uses a great deal of the body's large muscle groups.

As the weight drops down, bend at the knees and hips, going back into a half squat and swing the bell between the legs. As you straighten up, the bell is driven from the legs and body to be carried back to the raised position.

Throughout the motion, the back is kept straight. Try your best to also keep straight arms as you raise and lower the weight. Don't arch your back as the weight reaches the top – Keeping tight abdominals will assist in this.

One Arm Snatch

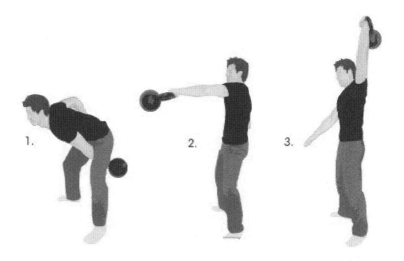

The one arm snatch is a favourite of mine because it utilises nearly every muscle in the body. It's also incredibly fun and there's something just very raw about it.

The one arm snatch should be considered an advancement of the one arm kettlebell swing, so I'd suggest becoming proficient at the above exercise first; with both arms as well as with one since you'll only be using the one arm here.

The difference between the snatch and the swing is that the snatch movement continues until the bell is in the overhead raised position. As usual, swing the bell from between your legs and as the bell raises, lead the motion with your elbow, as if you're about to elbow somebody taller than you in the face. When the bell is in front of your head, simply use a push or spear motion upwards with your arm to raise it to the overhead position. Hold for a beat and then from there, allow gravity to return the bell back to between the legs – Repeat.

The whole motion should be fluid and smooth.

It's important not to hold too tightly onto the weight or it could bang against your forearm in the raised position. A few too many of those and you'll give yourself a bruise.

Figure 8 Curl

This exercise is wonderful for improving coordination and balance as well as strengthening the core muscles. The figure 8 curl is only possible to perform using one kettlebell.

Begin in a half squat and using one hand, pass the weight through your legs and around the back of one knee where your free hand grabs the weight round the other side. From there, bring the weight round the front of your body and curl it up to your chest using a motion identical to a typical bicep curl. Allow the weight to drop down and pass through the legs again. This time, thread the bell round the back of the opposite knee where your free hand will again grasp the handle to bring round the front of your body and again curl up to your chest.

The bell threads between the legs in a figure of 8. The movement is fluid and controlled and should not require any great deal of skill.

As the kettlebell passes between the knees, ensure you bend them slightly along with your hips and use the straightening movement along with the generated momentum to power the curl.

Ensure the back is flat throughout the entire movement.

Squat and Press

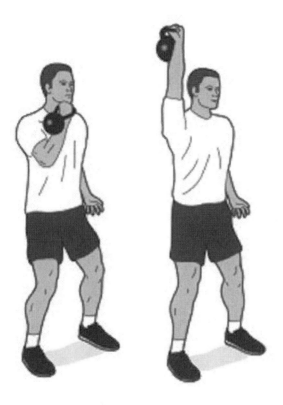

Unlike with the clean and press, with the squat and press the kettlebell remains in the racked position as in the diagram. This exercise works the majority of the body's large muscle groups.

Beginning from a half squat, clean the bell into the racked starting position as shown on the left. Lower yourself into a squat, taking care to go as deep as is comfortable (the deeper you go the more the glutes are incorporated). As you straighten your knees and hips, driving up through the feet, use the momentum to raise the weight above the head in an explosive motion. Control the downward movement of the weight back into the racked position. Then repeat.

Please ensure the bell is returned to the racked position *before* beginning the next squat otherwise the movement could cause you to lose balance.

Lunge and Press

The lunge and press is another exercise that will work a high number of large muscle groups.

Clean the kettlebell up and, if pressing with both hands then hold the weight in front of your chest with both hands. If you're pressing with single arms then clean the weight up into the racked position, ensuring to keep your elbow close into your body.

Lunge forward, bending at the front knee and lowering your rear knee under control towards the floor. As you lower the rear knee toward the floor, simultaneously press the bell straight up and above your head. Complete the manoeuvre by driving up from the front foot while also lowering the weight back toward your chest or racked position.

If pressing with a single arm then always lunge forward with the same leg that is performing the press.

When beginning, this exercise may involve a high level of concentration, skill and balance. It is advisable to begin with extremely light kettlebells. You will benefit from incredible improvements in motor skills by carrying out this exercise on a regular basis.

Keep both feet pointing forward throughout the motion, as well as a straight back and tight abdominals. Don't lunge further forward than is comfortable. If you're not well versed in lunging then please practice the exercise without the press incorporated into it. You can always add the press into subsequent training sessions in order to add another element of difficulty.

Bodyweight Circuits

There are so many different bodyweight exercises that are possible that you'll never find yourself becoming bored with them. However, due to the vast choice available, for HIIT purposes the emphasis should always be placed on selecting those exercises that work the larger muscle groups the hardest. These will predominantly be the legs and core. By selecting exercises that target these areas, you are certain to create a fast lactic acid build up in order to achieve the desired training effect.

These exercises can in the majority of instances be carried out with no equipment. So you can train at home, in the park or in the gym if you choose.

Also, there's nothing stopping you from mixing in these exercises with the above kettlebell exercises for added variation.

These exercises are intense. If doing bodyweight circuits, I highly recommend you pay extra attention to the *dynamic stretching* section below. Many of the bodyweight circuit exercises, particularly the jumping based exercises are by their very nature explosive. Dynamic stretching beforehand will serve you extremely well in preventing any muscle strains during the exercise. The first few times you carry these out, you're going to feel extremely sore for a couple days afterwards. For this reason, I also suggest you pay extra care to carry out static stretches (see *Post*

Workout Stretching) as well as these will partly mitigate the soreness over the following days.

As stated earlier – There are reasons many people associate bodyweight circuits as well as kettlebell exercises with the Tabata protocol. It's because they are extremely intense. This being so makes them perfect for us and what we're trying to achieve.

If you're using the Tabata protocol with bodyweight circuits then you should use the 10 second recovery period to shake yourself loose and to take in a few deep breaths. By no means should you begin light jogging around the room as you'll regret it come the next high intensity interval.

If you're using a HIIT protocol and therefore longer recovery periods then there are still many things you can do between high intensity bodyweight circuit exercises. Jogging on the spot or around the room, a brisk walk or very light skipping are all ideal.

Below are a selection of bodyweight circuit exercises along with brief instructions. Select the best few for yourself. As always, if in any doubt, a trainer at your local gym can show you the proper technique. Failing that, there are many online videos available that clearly demonstrate safe and effective technique.

High Knees

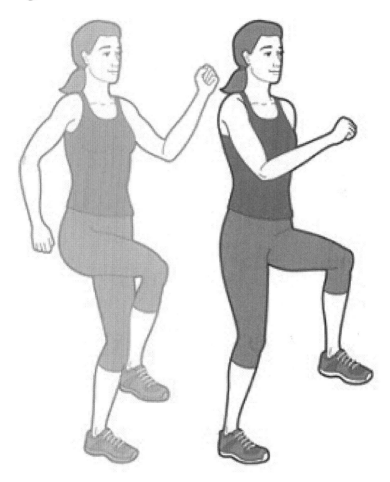

These are an ideal exercise to start with since they are low impact compared to many of the alternatives, therefore they can be treated as part of the warm up before really going all out with the subsequent exercises.

High knees are fairly self-explanatory. The technique is effectively a jogging on the spot movement while concentrating on bringing your knees higher than feels natural.

High knees can be made more intense by speeding up the activity while also raising your knees even higher.

Squat Thrusts / Burpees

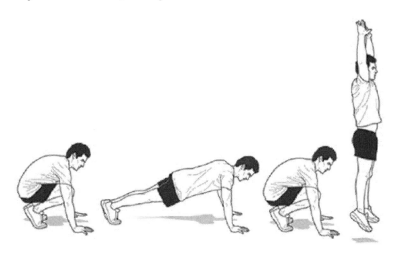

We'll cover both squat thrusts and burpees in this section since there's only one addition from the squat thrust to turn the exercise into a burpee. This exercise works practically every muscle in the body and so will exhaust you quickly.

From a crouched position, place your weight on your hands and shoot your legs straight behind so you end up in the press up position. From here you have the option of adding a press up into the exercise if you choose. Next, shoot your legs back up toward your hands so you're back in the original crouched position. To perform a squat thrust - Simply stand up then crouch back down again and repeat. If you're doing burpees, then instead of simply standing up, jump up into the air in an explosive thrust, stretching your hands up as you do before landing on your feet and returning to the crouch. Repeat.

Squat Jumps

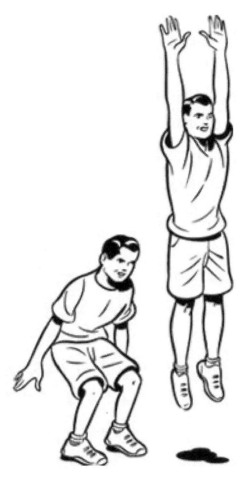

This exercise demonstrates just why dynamic stretching is recommended prior to beginning your session (see section on *Dynamic Stretching* below).

Keep your feet at a shoulder width distance. Control the lowering into the squat and try gain some depth. The more depth you get, the more the powerful glutes are utilised in the explosive movement during the upwards motion. Push through your heels as hard as you can, leaping into the air and stretching your arms to the sky. Keep a flat back throughout and ensure a comfortable landing on the toes.

Many people prefer pointing the arms to the floor as this makes balancing easier. To make the move more advanced therefore, you can point the arms to the sky. You can also concentrate on driving a greater push up through the feet and gaining a higher leap to make the exercise even more intense. It's possible to incorporate a sideward jump into the manoeuvre, jumping wider and wider as you get more used to the variation.

Box Jumping

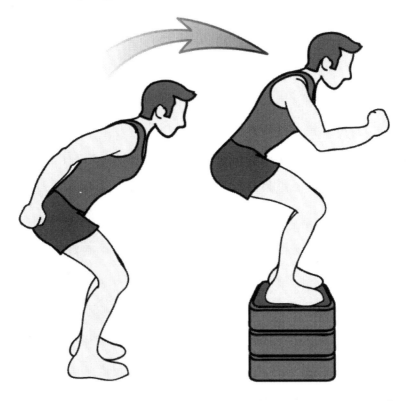

This is one of the few exercises where you need a minimal amount of equipment. All gyms will have boxes which you can stack on top of each other. Otherwise a ledge, bench, high step or suitable wall will work just as well. I know a couple of people who've assembled their own jump boxes using wood from the local DIY store.

With box jumps, you'll find it easier if you don't squat down further than what is necessary. Instead use your arms in a swinging motion to gain momentum for the upward thrust while pushing up through your toes. Bring your knees toward your chest while in the air and keep a flat back.

Once on the box, step up to a fully straightened position, gather your balance for a beat then simply jump backwards the way you came. Repeat.

Keep your knees wide apart (shoulder width) during the entire movement. If you feel them collapsing inwards, then position your feet slightly closer together.

An advanced variation of this exercise is to jump fully over the box, turn around and repeat. You can also carry out the exercise with weights in your hands, which will place even more emphasis on the legs. You can even eliminate the arm swinging motion to force the legs to be even more explosive. Finally, you can raise the height of the box to make the jumps even more intense.

Mountain Climbers

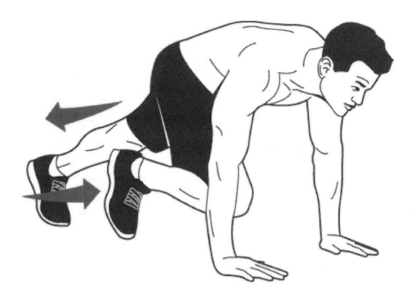

Begin in a peaked push up position with your glutes pointing in the air, placing all weight on your hands. Your arms should be fully vertical throughout the entire exercise with the shoulder fully over the hands. Bring one foot in front of the other so that you're in a comfortable starting position. When ready, switch the position of your legs by utilising a single shifting movement. Repeat again and again in rhythmical fashion. Your hips will bob up and down slightly, which is ok. Once you find your rhythm, feel free to increase the speed to make the exercise more intense.

Concentrate on maintaining a nice breathing rhythm.

Lunge Jumps

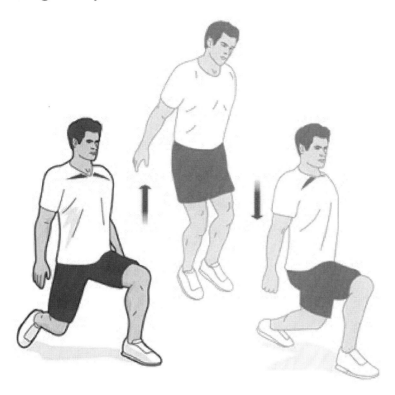

From a standing position, take a large step forward, bending the front knee and dropping the rear knee toward the floor, but not touching it. Jump up through your front foot in an explosive motion and switch legs in mid-air so that your rear leg moves to the front. When the trailing leg reaches the rear, drop the knee toward the floor and repeat.

This move should be carried out on the spot. Ensure you keep a straight back throughout, which should be kept in a straight line above the rear knee.

This exercise is advanced and is excellent for improving balance and coordination. If you feel you lack the balance required then the exercise can be made easier simply by eliminating the leg switching movement. This will still give you an incredible training effect. To make more intense, hold some light weights in your hands.

Tuck Jumps

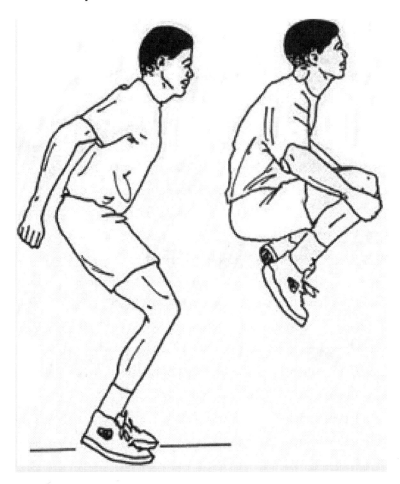

Tuck jumps are similar to squat jumps. The only difference is that this time the aim is to bring the knees in toward the chest before landing. Try and maintain a deep squat just like with squat jumps.

Lateral Box Jumps

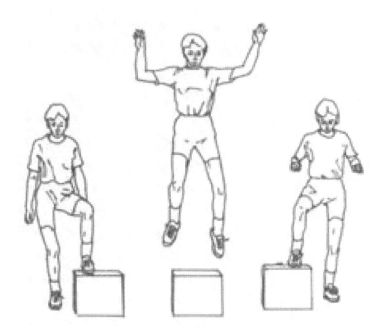

All that's required is a box. There are several variations to this exercise and I hope you'll try them all.

First – Standing to the side of the box, with both feet on the floor, carry out a high jump to the side and landing on top of the box. Jump off the opposite side and repeat in the other direction.

Second – To make the exercise a little harder, you'll be performing a full side jump over the box. Standing to the side of the box, with both feet on the floor, carry out a high jump to the side and fully over the box, landing on the other side. Repeat in the opposite direction.

Third – As in the picture and to make the exercise harder still, you'll be performing the jump using the power from only one leg from a raised position on the box. Push down through the foot of the raised leg in an explosive manoeuvre and land on the opposite side with your other foot on the box ready to take off for the next repetition.

In all exercises you can use your arms to gather momentum and swing yourself over. In the third exercise, you'll find this necessary.

You can make the exercises more intense by raising the height of the box or by speeding up the jumps.

Summary

As you've seen, there are many potential HIIT training modes and within each mode there are modifications you can make in order to increase the intensity incrementally and to ultimately provide a superior training effect.

I understand that most people, myself included, will decide upon their favourite training mode and carry out the vast majority of training within that discipline. Of course that's fine but I'd like you to consider a few points with regards to *cross-training*.

Cross-training refers to training utilising a multi-aspect approach. For example; running on Monday, weights on Tuesday and flexibility training on both Monday and Tuesday would be considered just one example of *cross-training* and is highly recommended for everybody no matter what their training goals may be.

However, keeping in scope with this book, I would like to talk about cross-training with regards to cardio based exercises only – Exercises where we can utilise the HIIT principles.

Each training mode, whether you're doing HIIT or CT, will utilise specific muscles and nerves in different ways, with different movements, at different frequencies, at different angles, with different ranges of motion at the joints, with a varying degree of force. By carrying out exercise on a bike or rower, you may feel like you're exercising your running muscles, but this will not in fact be giving you the same kind of training as running actually does – Not any more than exercising on a bike or rower would be considered the same kind of training as skipping, swimming or swinging kettlebells.

Each training mode is highly specific. If you don't believe me then simply ask a triathlete if he or she thinks that spending hours in the pool or hours running helps them with their cycling. On the contrary - The interesting element with the triathlon is that by spending time training with either of the three disciplines (swimming, cycling, running), they are actually counteracting what is needed with the other two. Consider that just one training adaptation is the growth of new blood vessels, capillaries in particular which transport fuel, water and oxygen to the working muscles. If you predominantly carry out cycling then the bulk of these new capillaries will be created in the lower extremities. Even though the individual may be considered cardiovascularly fit in an overall context, he may well then have difficulties when switching from cycling to swimming, or from swimming to running.

I'm not telling you this to put you off HIIT cross-training. In fact quite the contrary, I realise the majority of people reading this book will not be triathletes, but I want you to realise there are physiological forces at work that are not yet fully understood and that we should be encouraging partaking in a range of training modes for an all-round better fitness.

Taking the principle of the triathlete a little further – If you are in fact a professional or recreational athlete then for me to suggest that you take part in activities that are not sport specific to you is absurd. Athletes should always consider the principle of the specificity of training – If you want to be a good runner then run. If you want to be a good cyclist then cycle. If you want to be a good football player then practice HIIT while using the one training mode that most closely resembles football.

It's fairly well known in sport science that achieving a good aerobic or anaerobic base is general, in that there are indeed crossover benefits from improving cardiovascular capacity whether on a treadmill or bicycle. Anybody can improve their VO2 max whether skipping or swimming and likewise, anybody can lose weight or push back their anaerobic threshold whether stair climbing or doing bodyweight circuits. But going beyond a *good* base then cardiovascular modes should be as specific to the athlete's sport as is possible.

To reiterate – At novice stages, all training modes can improve general fitness. However, as one progresses, then all training attributes will improve in ways specific to that mode.

Of course if you're an athlete then you're likely to already know the importance of sport-specific training and it would be pointless for a professional runner to start hitting the pool at 5am every morning in the hope it will improve his running performance.

So let's now consider the recreational exerciser, the young man who wants to get in shape, the lady who wants to tone up, the overweight teenager, the middle-aged man or woman who is only just getting back into fitness following a prolonged period of time being sedentary. These are the people I wrote this book for.

Though the science is far from definitive, there's a growing body of opinion that agrees that cross-training may be beneficial for a number of reasons.

The American Orthopaedic Society for Sports Medicine says that cross-training can provide a total body tune up. This is something you won't get from only concentrating on one type of activity.

Coming from a common-sense perspective, one can also envisage that cross-training, by randomly selecting from the large selection of HIIT modes above that this would prevent boredom and maintain exercise adherence. Not that HIIT is boring anyway, but you get the idea.

Another benefit is that by exercising a range of muscle groups in different ways alternatively, by choosing different HIIT modes, this may help the individual adapt quicker to new activities. This makes sense. If you're trained in a range of exercise modes then picking up a tennis racket for the first time in your life would be easier for you than if you only ever ran or cycled.

But the primary benefit to cross-training appears to be the reduction in overuse injuries. This is because cross-trainers are not using the same muscles and the same joints in the same way, every time they train.

By spreading the quantity of cumulative stress over a greater number of muscles and joints then individuals can reasonably expect to be able to exercise for longer periods, for greater intensities and much later into their lives. By concentrating on a single activity for years on end, one can expect an increased likelihood of excessively overloading and gradually wearing down vulnerable parts of the body such as the knees, shoulders, hips, ankles, elbows and back. It's important to realise that all cardio exercises, which keep us fit and healthy, utilise repetitive motions of these vulnerable parts. In fact for this very reason, it's even more important for people, once reaching middle-age to cross-train. And this becomes even more crucial still if the individual is particularly prone to injuries or is slow to recover from previous training sessions.

The aim of any training regime, no matter who you are or what your goals may be should be to "shock the body," to create a condition where the body needs to develop, to stress the body in order for it to adapt. By engaging in the same training mode every single time you lace up your training shoes, your body will rapidly become accustomed to the training regime.

Sure you can regularly increase the intensities and ramp up the difficulty of your HIIT protocols, but why not speed up and maximise on your gains by also alternating HIIT modes? By varying HIIT modes regularly you can expect to trigger even faster and more satisfying results.

And in the process, you maximise the chances of remaining fit and healthy, with the capacity to carry out HIIT into the latter stages of your life.

HIIT Best Practices

Before we begin our HIIT session, it's important that our muscles are prepared for the high intensity that's to come. Remember that HIIT is intensive. It's not wise to begin a HIIT session with an all-out sprint. It's far safer to build up to the high intensity periods in a safe, effective and gradual way. Because of this, it's advised that HIIT participants undergo a short pre-workout routine.

Once the session is finished, there should also be a managed, safe and effective post workout routine to ensure a speedier recovery for the next workout.

Below is a checklist of what should be carried out during an entire HIIT session. We'll cover each area now:

- Warm Up
- Dynamic Stretching
- Have A Workout Structure And Target
- Start Low And Build Up
- Ensure Readiness For The Next Interval
- Warm Down
- Post Workout Stretching
- Resting

Warm Up

If I choose to do a HIIT sprint workout in the local park, then it's a 7 minute walk from my front door. This walk is an essential part of my warm up.

As soon as I arrive at the park, I begin a slow jog. This jog lasts for around 3 minutes until I reach the track. I have a tree which marks the spot where I begin my dynamic stretching routine (see immediately below).

By this point I've had a nice gradual warm up, oxygenated blood is already flowing at a faster rate around my body ready to give energy and oxygen to my muscles when the real work begins. If the blood is not already flowing at an increased rate when I begin my high intensity intervals then oxygen and energy cannot get to where they're needed quick enough. This is why you tire out and fatigue quickly when you don't warm up.

To reiterate – If you work at 100% intensity without having gradually increased your heart rate, then you will not have adequately prepared your heart and lungs to deliver oxygenated blood to your muscles, which in turn will not have been prepared to receive it. This will result in a sluggish training session where you'll be performing far below your capabilities.

A warm up also oils your joints in preparation for the work ahead. It does this by distributing synovial fluid, a natural lubricant. This will help prevent an injury.

Warming up enhances the transmission of nerve impulses, helping you think, act and react quicker. This is the reason you don't think clearly when you just wake up, because your nerves are cold.

While it's perhaps best as well as most convenient to warm up using a mode specific to the impending HIIT session, it's not absolutely essential. If the HIIT workout is sprinting, then jogging is the obvious warm up. If cycling, then an easy cycle with low resistance is obvious since you'll already be sat on the bike. Likewise with rowing or any other mode you choose. Moving the muscles, the legs in particular in a way specific to the approaching workout makes complete sense for reasons of specificity.

If you're carrying out a kettlebell or bodyweight circuit session then yes, it is possible to carry out the forthcoming exercises with less intensity, using lower weights and without incorporating a full range of motion – A half squat with no weights for example. But my personal preference would be to utilise a treadmill, rower or cycle ergometer rather than an easier version of bodyweight circuits.

Once the warm up has been completed, then move quickly on to some dynamic stretching.

Dynamic Stretching

Remember physical education or gym classes back at school when you used to always carry out a bunch of static stretches before the real work began? Well this is an example of an unnecessary practice that is in the national psyche simply through habit (much like CT actually). Not only is a pre-workout static stretch not necessary, it is actually potentially dangerous.

To clear up any confusion, static stretches are the most commonly used stretches that are held at a point of tension for around 10 – 15 seconds. We have been using them all our lives.

The reason we were always made to do static stretches pre-workout was to prevent injury. That was the only reason. However, studies have shown that there are no differences to the level of injuries sustained during the subsequent activity between groups that carry out pre-workout static stretches and those that don't.

In fact by giving cold muscles static stretches before your workout has even begun, you are in fact more likely to be injured during or after the activity than if you don't stretch. It's far easier to tear a cold muscle than a warmed up muscle due to it being less malleable. So you really don't need to bother wasting your time carrying out pre-workout static stretches, and that goes for the rest of your life, it's just not necessary.

However, *dynamic stretching* is another matter entirely. Dynamic stretches use controlled movements in order to improve range of motion, loosen up the muscles, increase the heart rate and body temperature as well as the blood flow around the body. In fact, incorporating dynamic stretching at this point in your HIIT session can be considered an extended part of your warm up.

Dynamic stretching is most effective when used prior to activities that involve explosive movements. For HIIT purposes, this would most likely encompass sprinting and jumping, though explosive bursts are possible in a range of other HIIT modes too. All professional and recreational sprinters and many middle and longer distance runners use dynamic stretches as an essential part of their pre-workout regime. Though personally I don't believe dynamic stretching is necessary for endurance athletes, since most sports involve short bursts of explosive activity, dynamic stretching proves useful for the vast majority of professional and recreational athletes. No matter what your present physical condition and no matter what your future goals may be – If you are utilising explosive body movements in your HIIT workouts, which I accept will be the case in the vast majority of instances, then I recommend you incorporate dynamic stretches into your sessions.

Dynamic stretching is used to its best effect when the movements are kept specific to the upcoming activity. For sprints you would mimic sprint movements and for jumps you would mimic jumping movements etc.

The idea is to start slowly, using a small range of motion and focusing on good form. After a set number of repetitions (usually a small number) and you feel the movements becoming easier, then you would gradually increase the range of motion as well as speed. The key is to keep the movements dynamic. At the further points of the larger movements made, the muscles are being stretched for a brief second (dynamically) and in a manner that will soon be occurring during the chosen activity.

For HIIT sprint and jumping workouts, particular emphasis should be placed on the hamstrings; a common area of straining (as we'll learn in the section entitled *HIIT Pitfalls*).

There is no requirement to spend a great deal of time carrying out dynamic stretches. You should spend only the amount of time required to bring your joints through the greater ranges of motion, thus stretching the muscles, for a small number of repetitions. Once you reach your full range of motion, ten repetitions are usually enough for most people to have dynamically stretched the targeted muscles. Although you should always use your own best judgement and listen to your body. There are many factors at play that could affect your state on the day and therefore how many repetitions you should carry out. Temperature, weather, surface, hydration, alertness, mood and time of day can all play a part and affect your flexibility at any given time. If in doubt, it's always preferential to carry out a few extra repetitions than too few and risk straining a muscle because you performed explosive movements on cold muscles that hadn't been fully mobilised and stretched.

As you may have already guessed, I'm a fan of getting in there and getting out. I like to get the greatest benefits from my workouts in the shortest possible time period. If you would prefer to spend more of your time carrying out an extended warm up (that was specific to your HIIT mode) then there will be a gradually diminished need to spend more time dynamic stretching. Likewise the same goes for the opposite – Since dynamic stretching utilises large movements of the body, which in some instances are quite intense as you're about to discover, if you would rather spend more time dynamic stretching, you can choose to shorten your warm up. As always, listen to your body and never go all out 100% for your high intensity interval until you're satisfied you are thoroughly prepared.

Now we'll take a look at a range of specific dynamic stretches.

Pike Stretch

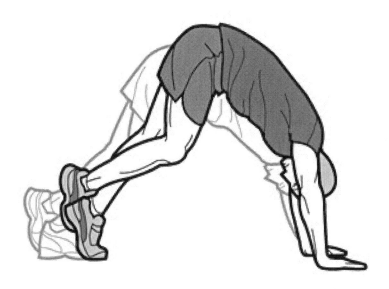

Target Muscles – Calf Muscles

I recommend beginning with the pike stretch since it's the least energetic of all the dynamic stretches we'll be covering. By starting with this one, you'll be able to build up to the more intense stretches below.

Begin with your hands and knees on the floor, then raise your hips into the air so your body is in the piked position as in the drawing. Take one foot from the ground and place it on the heel of the active (to be stretched) foot. Push down with your free foot so the heel of the active foot presses toward the ground. Hold for a second and release. Repeat.

If you're particularly flexible then you may not require the use of your free foot for pressing down the active foot.

To increase the intensity of the stretch, slide the feet further away from your hands. If you weren't already, you can also ensure your heel presses all the way to the ground.

Butt Kicks

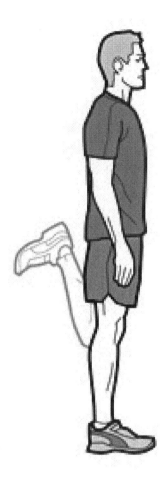

Target Muscles – Quadriceps

Stand tall and walk forward with an exaggerated back kicking motion with your heels moving toward your glutes. Increase the intensity by advancing to a slow jog, kicking higher and faster.

Leg Swings

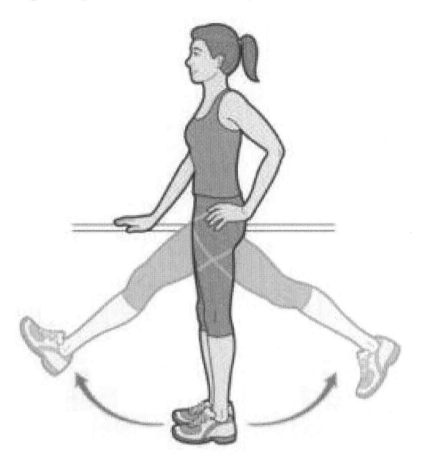

Target Muscles – Hip Flexors, Glutes, Hamstrings

Best used with a wall, tree or rail as a support.

The forward swing stretches the glutes and hamstrings, whereas the backward swing stretches the hip flexors.

The knees should be soft and not locked out. In fact the emphasis with the forward swing portion of this exercise should be placed on the glutes which means you don't need to be too concerned with keeping your knee overly straight – Hamstrings are secondary here and this provides a nice warm up for the straight leg raises (hamstrings) later on. During the backward phase of the swing, the knees will naturally bend regardless.

Begin slow with a small range of motion. Increase the intensity by speeding up the movement and increasing the range of motion.

Straight Leg Raises

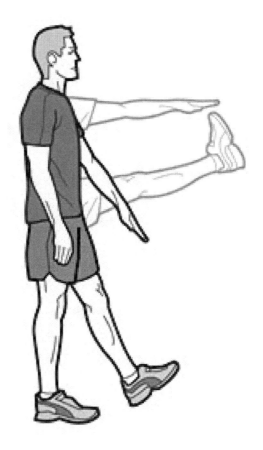

Target Muscles – Hamstrings, Calf Muscles

Unlike the compound stretch above, here we are primarily stretching the hamstrings, a crucially important area for dynamic stretching prior to sprinting or jumping.

Maintain a straight posture as you walk forward lifting your legs in the air. Ensure your knee remains as straight as possible as bending it in any way will shorten rather than lengthen the hamstrings which we are targeting here. By pointing the toes toward your head, the calf muscles will also be dynamically stretched. Look straight forward while carrying out the exercise as this will aid balance.

To advance this exercise, simply increase the speed or add a skipping motion instead of walking. The legs can also be raised higher.

Walking Lunges

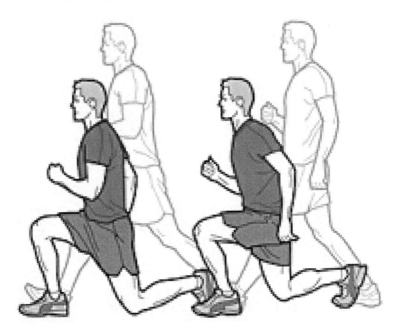

Target Muscles – Hip Flexors, Hamstrings, Quadriceps, Calf Muscles

Walking lunges are a mini-workout in themselves. For this reason they should be put at the end of your dynamic stretching routine when you'll be most warmed up and ready to begin your high intensity intervals.

This dynamic stretch also involves all the running muscles including the glutes if a slight modification is made.

Place your hands on your hips and step forward with one foot. Bend your front leg as you lower your back leg to the ground in a controlled manner. The front knee should not extend beyond the point of the toes and you should not allow your rear knee to touch the ground. Your body weight should be centred over the front leg and you use the same foot to push back up to a standing position. Now step through with your rear foot thus changing sides. Keep an upright posture throughout, pulling in your abdominals.

In order to add a stretch to your glutes - As you bring your rear leg forward, first raise the knee (of the rear leg) up to your chest. Clasp at the knee using both hands and pull the knee into your chest. You should feel the stretch in your glutes. Bring the leg down in front, going into your next lunge. This is in effect incorporating a standing knee raise to your lunges.

By now you should be thoroughly warmed-up, dynamically stretched and ready to begin your high intensity intervals. But remember to use your own best judgement. It may be an extremely cold day and if you're exercising outside, then you can always go back into a warm up and build up to the high intensity intervals.

Have A Workout Structure And Target

It would be beneficial to enter your training session with a HIIT protocol and mode in your head and therefore some sort of idea of any targets within that session. For example; how many high intensity intervals are you hoping to squeeze in? Will it be one more than during the previous workout? Will the high intensity periods be more intense or will the recovery periods be shorter?

I always like to know exactly what the coming workout has in store for me, then if I don't achieve my goals, I can beat myself up over it and make sure I achieve them the time after. I do this by analysing where I went wrong – Was I not properly hydrated? Did I not get enough sleep? Were the intervals too tough for me? Or was I just having a bad day?

I would also suggest making a record of your achievements at the end of your workout. The following could be useful; number of intervals, % of maximal heart rate, duration of high intensity periods, duration of recovery periods, HIIT mode.

By keeping a record of the above variables, improving on each subsequent training session can be an attainable target. If you intend on regularly alternating HIIT modes then it could be a while before returning to say rowing and remembering the exact protocol could be tricky.

Getting more specific - Let's take the example that you'll be carrying out HIIT running outside in the park, but feel free to modify accordingly depending on your chosen activity. I have to use some sort of an example here and I've chosen running outside as it's genuinely very popular.

It would be best to have a predetermined route planned out. So why not take a walk along your chosen path the day before your first session. Mark out where you'll begin your walk, where you'll start your light jog and your marker (tree, lamp post, trash can) for your first high intensity interval.

Then mark out the spot where this sprint will end and your recovery period will begin. This recovery period should be quite lengthy when starting out, maybe even up to 3 minutes in duration so have this pre-planned. Then locate your next landmark for your next high intensity interval.

I've found that this is so much easier if you have a circuit, such as a track around the outside of a park then you can use the same markers on each lap as your cue to change speed.

Of course, you can bypass using any markers at all if you use the Fartlek protocol and simply listen to your own body.

Start Low And Build Up

You need to think about your existing level of fitness.

Are you immediately ready to go for a full on HIIT session consisting of between 8 – 10 high intensity periods with only very short recovery periods? Or is your present fitness level a little more modest and you're in need of working up to the former?

Everybody has to start somewhere so don't fret if you're nervous about putting this book down and starting your first HIIT session.

If you're fit and confident, then you may as well dive straight in at the deep end and see how you get on with it. There's no way any number of all-out sprints interspersed with recovery periods will phase or harm you. Just make a note of your variables and try to advance yourself on the subsequent sessions.

For those starting with modest fitness, then this section is a little more for you.

If you're beginning from an extremely low cardio base, then I suggest taking at least two CT sessions first. If you're able to run, cycle, row etc for 30+ minutes at 70% maximal heart rate, then in my opinion, you're perfectly fine to jump straight into an easy interval training protocol at the very least.

While the Little Method is ideal for intermediates, there are always ways of manipulating an interval training protocol to suit outright beginners.

From a relative warm up intensity such as walking or light jogging, then injuries permitting, anybody no matter who they are will be able to increase the intensity to something higher than the warm up state. Bingo - Because as soon as you've done this, then as long as you return to a lower intensity then this can be considered interval training.

If your recovery intensity is 50 – 60% maximal heart rate (achievable for everybody) then raising that to 70 – 85% will be manageable by everybody too.

If you're intending on taking it easy during the first session, then 4 high intensity periods, at 30 seconds each will give you a feel for what it's all about. Judge for yourself, in the moment, how long the recovery periods should be and then take the next high intensity intervals when ready – An easy Fartlek protocol. All I do ask is that you record the variables and endeavour to smash them on each subsequent training session. Trust me, there's no better feeling than improving just that little bit with each subsequent training session and while you're still discovering exactly where your fitness or HIIT level is then these original *improvements* will come thick and fast. It's similar to beginning a strength training regime - Until you know what you're capable of lifting then there'll be much experimentation until you find the correct weights, with each exercise that you're capable of lifting between 6 – 8 times until you reach overload.

Though I will reiterate this here, as I have several times already – It's all about intensity. And I urge you to push yourself and see just what you're capable of achieving, rather than playing it safe. You may just surprise yourself.

Ensure Readiness For The Next Interval

Remember that a crucial part of HIIT is the recovery period. Don't assume that just because you're walking or cycling at an easy intensity and you're finding the intensity to be extremely easy that you're somehow not doing HIIT correctly. The recovery period is just as important as the high intensity period. The walks are just as important as the sprints. The cycling on minimal resistance is just as important as cycling on high resistance.

So ensure your recovery periods are sufficient enough to bring your heart rate down to a more relaxed state and your body feels prepared for the next high intensity interval. Throughout your HIIT session there'll be several high intensity-intervals that if you don't feel shattered after your first or second, you will do by the time you get to your fourth of fifth, eleventh or twelfth.

So enjoy the recovery periods and make full use of them. They're also the best opportunity you'll have to take a gulp of water – Which I recommend you do often.

Warm Down

Just as warming up at the beginning of a HIIT session is crucial, so is warming down at the end. This is something that many people don't know the significance of and the effects of not warming down can be debilitating.

When you exercise, you are increasing the flow of blood around your body. So if you exercise hard, and then come to a sudden stop, although you and your muscles have stopped working, your blood will still be flowing at this increased rate. Because of gravity, your blood will tend to pool in your legs. If blood is pooled sufficiently so that there's a reduction in return flow to the heart then your blood pressure can drop and you will become dizzy or possibly even faint. I'm sure you're aware of the feeling of having heavy legs after a run, maybe even for a couple of days afterwards? This could have been due to not warming down properly and experiencing the subsequent blood pooling.

By gradually lowering the intensity of your HIIT session then you can safely bring your heart rate back down to a more regular pace.

The way I do this is that after I've finished my final high intensity period, instead of walking like I would a usual recovery period, I will instead lightly jog for a couple of minutes. Afterwards I will continue with a walk for a few minutes after that.

This way my heart rate has been gradually returned to a more normal pace, even though my blood is still circulating in a high gear, my legs are still moving too.

Never will I collapse on a bench after an all-out sprint.

Post Workout Stretching

I mentioned "heavy legs" in the section above; the feeling of not being able to move your legs the day or two after your workout. This feeling can be prevented by warming down as we've already discussed and also by carrying out a thorough post workout stretch.

When you carry out exercise, you are contracting your muscles, often with extreme force. Contracting is another word for shortening. If you don't stretch your muscles after you've been repeatedly shortening them during your workout then trust me, you'll know about it in the morning as you'll feel extremely stiff. You need to bring your muscles back to their pre-workout length by stretching them.

Post workout would also be a good time to try and *improve* your flexibility, by stretching perhaps a little deeper and for longer. These types of stretches are known as *developmental stretches* as they work on increasing your flexibility and not merely returning your muscles to their original length. Post workout is the safest and most effective time to carry out developmental stretches since you'll be thoroughly warmed up and your muscles will be the most pliable. If you already do, or intend to carry out a lot of HIIT after reading this book then developmental stretches should be a regular part of your post workout routine as they will help to improve your posture, decrease the chances of muscle cramping and will even lessen the chances of injury. The most common form of injury sustained by sprinters are hamstring strains (see the section on *HIIT Pitfalls* below as we go into this in detail) and so developmental stretches which target the hamstrings are particularly important for us.

Developmental stretches are similar to the usual static stretches we've been using all our lives. With a static stretch, the stretch is held for around 10 – 15 seconds at a point where the tension is felt. At the point in time where you feel the tension diminish - the stretch is developed further by going deeper into it and holding the position for around 30 seconds. As you sink further into the stretch, breathe out gently through your mouth. Once you feel the tension diminish once again, you can then go even further into the stretch. As you go deeper into the stretch, ensure you do so in a slow and controlled manner. Remember that the idea is to *feel* the tension otherwise you are not actually stretching the muscle. If you feel the tension too much so that it becomes uncomfortable then ease yourself out a little until it feels more bearable.

You should carry out a range of stretches on all the major muscles of the legs as well as the upper body, as don't forget, we also use the arms a great deal while running and using other modes of HIIT. While you can perform developmental stretches on any muscle, I feel the most important area for HIIT purposes are the hamstrings which also happens to be an area where too many people suffer from inflexibility. I will reiterate - It is advisable to at least carry out static stretches on all the main muscle groups immediately after your warm down. But if you decide to only carry out developmental stretches in one area, then this area should be the hamstrings.

Below are diagrams as well as instructions for carrying out a range of important stretches – beginning with the hamstrings, although please feel free to skip this part if you're fully aware about how these stretches are carried out. Explanations on how to develop each stretch further will also be given. In most instances, I give two variations of each stretch and you should carry out the stretch you prefer and feel you're getting the most benefit from. However, as always, alternating your stretches every few HIIT sessions will provide additional benefits.

Lying Hamstring Stretch

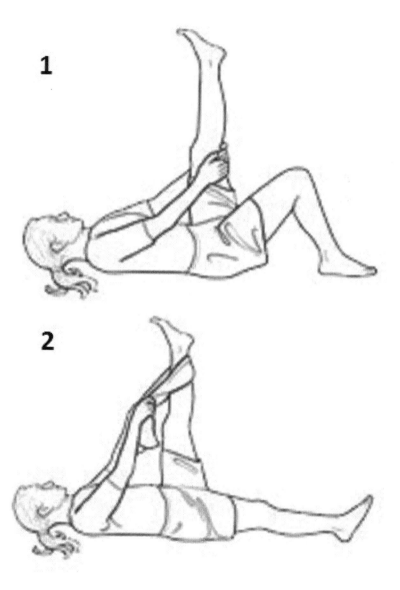

1

2

1. The lying hamstring stretch is carried out on each leg individually. Lie down with your back flat on the ground and raise one leg, taking hold behind the knee with your hands.

2. By bending the knee of your free leg you'll take pressure off your back.

3. Gently pull the leg towards yourself until you feel the stretch.

4. Ensure you keep the knee as straight as possible but not locked. You will feel a natural tendency to bend the knee, which will lessen the stretch – Try and avoid that.

5. If you're developing hamstring flexibility as suggested then when tension is no longer felt (20 – 30 seconds), ease the leg closer toward your chest until you feel new tension.

6. Repeat as necessary and then change legs.

7. Image 2 shows the use of a towel which may be used if you can't reach your knee.

Standing Hamstring Stretch

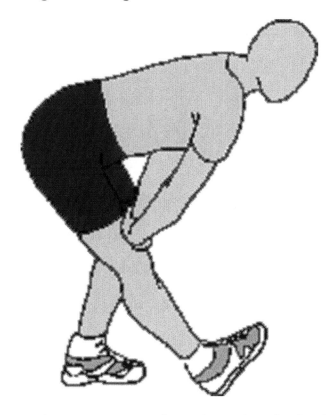

I'm sure the vast majority of people reading this book are familiar with this stretch. The standing hamstring stretch will yield the same results as the above lying hamstring stretch except by raising the toes of the leg being stretched, you can also gain a stretch on the calf muscles.

In order to develop further, simply lower your chest further toward the straightened leg, ensuring to keep the knee straight but not locked and your back straight. You can also slide the foot in closer toward your bent leg to deepen the stretch.

Standing Quadriceps Stretch

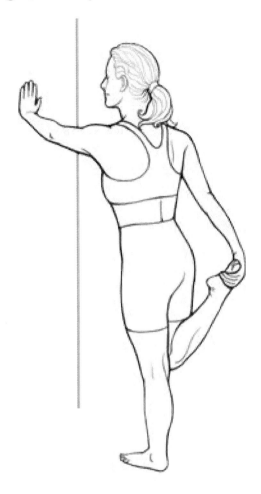

Balance yourself against a wall with one hand. Use your other hand to clasp the foot or ankle of the corresponding leg. Pull your foot toward your glutes until you feel the stretch in your quadriceps. You can increase this stretch by pulling your foot even closer to your glutes. If you're not feeling a deep enough stretch then try the method below.

Hip Flexor / Quadriceps Stretch

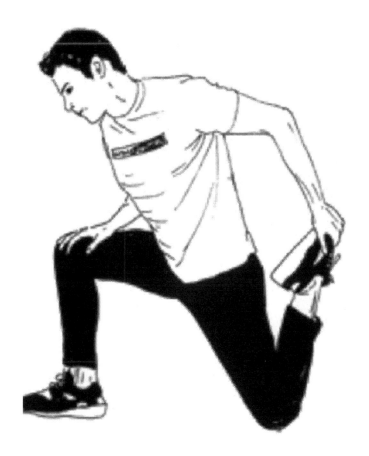

I will warn you that this stretch is deep. But it gets the job done. Not only does this stretch out your quadriceps extremely well, but also your illopsoas muscles which are the strongest of your hip flexors.

Kneel on the floor with one knee in front of the other. Bend the knee of your rear leg and clasp your foot with the corresponding hand. This may require balance so you may use a chair or wall to stabilise yourself. Be careful not to place too much weight on the knee – Leaning forward will take the weight off or you can place a towel between the knee and the floor. Once you're in position, simply push out your hips to feel the stretch in your hip flexors and quadriceps. You can develop the stretch by pushing your hips out further or by stepping forward gradually with your front foot.

Calf Stretch

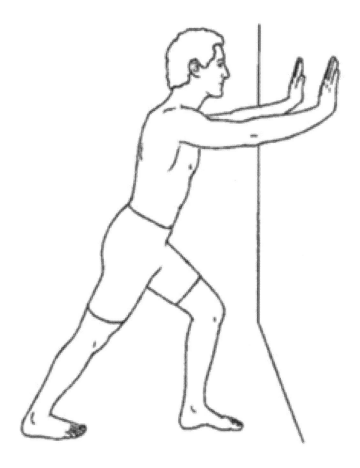

This is the classic calf muscle stretch I'm sure you've been using since you were a child. While you don't require a wall as illustrated in the drawing, using one will enable you to maintain a better balance. Ensure both feet point forwards and keep your rear foot flat against the floor. By sliding back the rear foot you decrease the angle between the toes and the shin, gradually lengthening the muscle in the back of the leg and increasing the tension of the stretch. Your rear heel may feel the natural tendency to rise up from the ground, but it's important to keep it flat. As with all developmental stretches, when you feel the tension wane, gradually increase the tension (in this case by sliding the rear foot further back) and hold for another 30 seconds.

Soleus Stretch

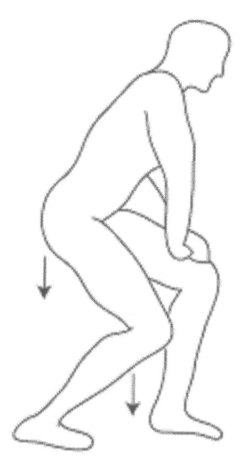

The soleus muscle runs deeper to the calves and connects to the heel. Many runners often find the soleus becomes tight, causing discomfort and it's thought that a tight soleus muscle may also be a contributing factor toward Achilles tendonitis (see *HIIT Pitfalls* for more on this). Despite this, it's not an area we often stretch, probably because we were never taught how to do it. Yet stretching the soleus is used as a preventative measure from Achilles tendonitis.

To carry out this stretch, the angle of the ankle joint between the toes and shin must be reduced. Unlike when stretching the calves however, when stretching the soleus, the knee is bent, in order to take the calf out of the stretch.

As in the diagram, the front leg is used for stabilisation. Bend the rear knee, ensuring you're narrowing the angle of the ankle joint. You'll feel the stretch at the back of your leg just above the heel.

To develop this stretch, simply lower your thighs closer to the ground as in the diagram, thus further decreasing the angle of the ankle joint.

This stretch is deep. I suggest you come out from the stretch slowly.

Alternative Soleus Stretch

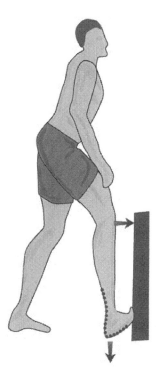

As an alternative to the above, you can simply use a wall, lamp post or pillar/post at the gym to stretch the soleus.

Plant the heel on the floor with your toes reaching upward against the wall for support. Move your knee towards the wall, thus reducing the angle at the ankle and stretching the muscle.

To develop further, simply move your knee closer to the wall.

This is a deep stretch that you will *feel*. When finished, ensure you relax out from it slowly.

Triceps Stretch

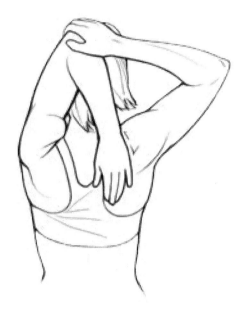

We need to also incorporate a number of upper body stretches in order to promote all over flexibility and good health. Let's not forget that we also use our arms when performing a large range of HIIT modes.

To carry out this upright triceps stretch, raise your arm above your head and bend at the elbow so that your hand presses against the top of your back. With your opposing hand, gently pull your elbow behind your head, feeling the hand of your stretched arm run slowly down your back.

To develop, pull further on the elbow, feeling the hand run slowly down the back.

Pectoralis Stretch

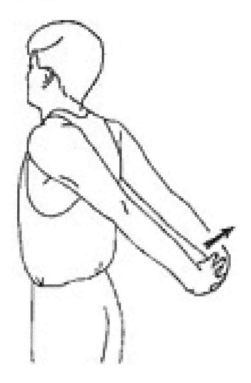

When sprinting, the upper portion of the pectorals is used to propel the arms forward, while the lower portion is used to drive them back. If you'll be carrying out sprinting yourself, which I hope you will be, then your chest will be working in overdrive. Therefore it's essential you pay attention to stretching out the pectorals, which you can do with this stretch, which also stretches the biceps.

Clasp your hands behind your back and pull them away. Keep soft elbows while carrying out this stretch.

To develop, simply work on pulling your arms further from the body.

Advanced Pectoralis / Front Deltoids Stretch

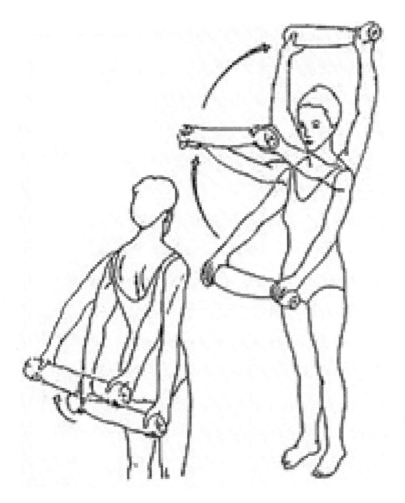

This stretch for the pectorals, front deltoids and biceps is advanced. If you stretch too deep too soon then you risk discomfort at the very least. However, this is a great stretch which you should want in your repertoire following any sprint session where the arms are used explosively.

Using a resistance band or failing that, a towel – Start with a wide grip, about one and a half shoulder widths on the towel in front of you. Raise your arms over your head and bring the towel down behind your back. When you feel the stretch – Stop. Wait until the tension wanes and then move the towel further down towards your lower back until you find a new area of tension and hold as necessary. This way you stretch both heads of the pectoralis major responsible for propulsion.

To develop further, simply narrow the grip on the towel and begin the stretch again.

Resting

There is a difference between inactivity and resting. Being inactive refers to spending your free time lying on the couch and generally being lazy. Whereas resting refers to quality time your body is using to repair, regenerate, readjust and evolve following a workout.

Resting is just as important as the workout itself as it's during the rest period that the body undergoes positive changes. And don't forget, it's during the rest stage that the magic of EPOC comes into play. It's due to EPOC that your body is still burning fat at an elevated rate for 48 hours post HIIT.

Just to clarify, by *rest* I'm not referring to the recovery periods during your HIIT session but instead to your rest days between HIIT sessions. Ideally you should carry out a HIIT session every other day, with a rest from HIIT in the days between.

I know it may be tempting to carry out two consecutive days of HIIT but I would strongly advise against it. Instead what you should do is consider your overall aims and goals. What are your reasons for undertaking HIIT sessions?

Are you strapped for time and in great need for the most time efficient fitness regime in existence? Are you looking simply to maintain your present physical condition? Or are you on a mission to lose a lot of weight and perhaps gain muscle too?

If the latter, then you should incorporate HIIT sessions between strength training sessions, perhaps at your local gym. Since there's the obvious requirement for rest and recovery days between strength sessions, then having a HIIT session on your "off" days would be ideal. Strength training and HIIT utilise different physiological systems and so you can naturally work one while resting the other alternately. Although strength training is beyond the scope of this book, this author does recommend it for everybody especially if you want to lose weight - Promoting muscle growth further aids fat loss. In addition you'll benefit from an increased resting metabolism as well as increased bone, muscle, ligament and tendon strength. Indeed, whatever your goals, strength training and HIIT complement each other perfectly.

If you do undertake both a HIIT and strength training regime then it's still crucial you take a minimum of one rest day per week for recovery. Any good trainer at your gym will be able to design a training programme for you based solely on your own aims and wishes, ensuring you incorporate adequate rest days between, depending on your present fitness. In addition, you'll need to ensure you're taking in adequate nutrition to support a training regime that's this intense on the body.

If at this stage in time strength training doesn't interest you, then every second day at minimum will be a rest and recovery day. If you have the urge to take part in something active then of course there is no problem with that. However I would refrain from partaking in all-out high intensity activity and opt for something slightly more leisurely. The best thing about HIIT is that it results in superior benefits and all in the least amount of time invested – Any extra vigorous cardio activity is unnecessary.

Getting More From HIIT

For this short section we're going to ignore all the other protocols and just concentrate on HIIT and on making HIIT even more advanced. We've covered all the basics including how beginners should take to their first few workouts. Now we're going to concentrate on those more advanced participants who really want to push themselves to see what they're capable of.

Following on from the last point in the above section, you may well be truly encouraged by your early progress, in fact I can assure you that this will happen. But rather than deciding to take more HIIT sessions in order to build on your progress, what I instead recommend you do is to increase the workload during your existing HIIT sessions. Remember that you will always need your rest days to maximise your gains.

You can increase your workload and make each individual HIIT session more intense via the following methods:

- If your HIIT sessions are not currently stretching for a duration of 30 minutes then you can increase the number of high intensity intervals (and by default the recovery periods too), effectively making for a longer HIIT session. Remember that there's no need to extend your HIIT session to beyond 30 minutes.

- Increase the intensity of the high intensity period (if not already at 100% of your maximal heart rate).
- This should be the most important factor; decrease the duration of the recovery period, making the entire session more intense. This should also enable you to fit in extra high intensity periods into your 30 minute session.
- Use gradients for your high intensity intervals by sprinting or cycling up hills. Increase any resistance of cardio equipment or add weights to bodyweight circuits as necessary.
- Finally, you can use one of the alternative HIIT modes as mentioned earlier to add variety and further shock your body.

Simply by phasing in these new elements over time, you'll be gradually making your HIIT session more intensive, keeping things interesting which is always recommended and you'll be exploiting your gains too.

You may have noticed that I did not add that you could "increase the length of your high intensity period." Can you guess why this is?

The reason is that if you're capable of increasing the length of your high intensity period then you're clearly not working hard enough. The aim is quality not quantity. If you're thinking to yourself that you could run for an extra five seconds at your fastest speed, then you clearly haven't been going all out at 100% up until now. The aim is to work as hard as you can, not for as long as you can - This element to HIIT is crucial.

Just to reiterate the above point and to really drill this home as it really is important; you need to set the high intensity interval period so that you really are working as hard as you're capable. The amount of time this takes is not really the issue, since if you're running, cycling or rowing as hard or as fast as you can, you will naturally fatigue within 10 – 30 seconds anyway. If you're able to sprint, cycle or row for any more than this amount of time, then you really do need to increase the intensity.

The amount of time it takes you to fatigue and require an urgent rest period will of course be different for everybody and there are many variables at play; your individual fitness, HIIT experience, which interval you're presently on, what your activity is, how you're feeling on that particular day as well as external weather conditions will all have an effect. This is why I'm very broad where I say that you'll naturally fatigue within 10 – 30 seconds. The amount of time is irrelevant as long as you do indeed work at as high an intensity as possible and you do indeed fatigue, this is all that really matters.

HIIT Nutrition

I'm sure you've read so many contradicting articles with regards to exercise nutrition that it's hard to know what to believe. Even much of the scientific research is contradictory.

The fact of the matter is that when it comes to fitness, the right diet for you will be different to what is right for somebody else. This is because the best diet for the individual is specific to their own aims and goals. The diet of somebody wishing to maintain present fitness levels would be different from somebody who wished to lose weight, which likewise would differ from someone who wanted to gain muscle. So when considering diet and nutrition, it's always important to consider your own reasons for engaging in HIIT to begin with.

Then you have to consider the very real fact that eating patterns for HIIT participants differ greatly from the eating patterns of CT participants. Or at least they really should differ, but that all depends on whether or not the participant has been given the correct information in the first place.

As you'll well know by now – HIIT is a completely different animal to CT. HIIT utilises additional physiological pathways that CT does not.

Let's consider CT for a minute. Although it's possible to find scientific literature that disagrees with the current consensus on nutrition, when partaking in say an hour of CT, the bulk of the literature is consistent. Let's also take the primary motivation for CT – Weight loss. If the participant wishes to lose weight with an hour of running on a treadmill at 70 – 75% maximal heart rate, then the advice is to arrive at the gym in a fasted state. If the body's supply of glycogen is depleted, or nearly depleted, then the body will be forced to tap into fat stores by oxidising free fatty acids for fuel. The result is weight loss from the CT session. If the participant steps onto the treadmill having in the last hour eaten a bowl full of porridge or oatmeal then before the body can access the free fatty acids, it would first have to use the ample supply of glycogen that came from the carbohydrates in the porridge.

Of course the above is a simplistic view of things. The body's muscles and tissues will in fact be utilising fuel from carbohydrates, fat and protein simultaneously, though in different proportions and dependent on the exercise intensity and muscle glycogen supply.

As a general rule of thumb – The muscles utilise a higher proportion of fuel from fat during exercise up to around 80% maximal heart rate, fasted state dependent. Once the exercise becomes more intense, then the body needs a more immediate source of fuel, something that does not require such long and complicated chemical reactions such as when breaking down free fatty acids. This fuel that is more easily obtainable comes from carbohydrates. In fact, at high intensities (85 – 100% maximal heart rate), such as during HIIT, barely any fat is utilised as fuel during the workout.

So if weight loss is the goal during a CT workout, then you need to exercise in a fasted, or near fasted state at an intensity of 75% maximal heart rate for around 45 – 60 minutes. *Fasted state* could refer to exercising before breakfast or having not eaten for 3 – 4 hours.

I can sense alarm bells going off in the heads of my readers. I can imagine that many of you are wondering, "Hang on – So you don't burn fat during HIIT? Then why am I doing this?"

My response to the above query would be to remind you of EPOC. Realise that the vast majority of fat burning from a HIIT workout occurs *after* the training session and not during.

In fact, for our CT treadmill runner, as soon as he returns home, his fat burning will slow to a pace more resembling the great masses of the population. But for a HIIT participant, his fat oxidation will continue to be elevated for 48 hours post HIIT.

The other luxury afforded to the HIIT over the CT participant is that with HIIT there's no requirement to exercise in a fasted state. Due to HIIT intensities being too high for fat oxidation to take place in any meaningful way during the workout, it would be pointless exercising in a fasted state. In fact, fasted state exercise with HIIT would most likely even be detrimental to the quality of the workout and would even result in muscle wasting which goes completely against what you should be trying to achieve, no matter what your aims.

At high intensities, glycogen from carbohydrate is the preferred source of fuel. Without it then you'd be in for an extremely sluggish HIIT session.

My advice – Eat something, preferentially complex carbohydrate based within two hours prior to a HIIT workout.

There's no need to make things any more complicated than the above paragraph. And that holds true no matter what your aims, goals or objectives may be for partaking in HIIT.

The above is one reason why HIIT workouts are short. Once glycogen supply runs out, then muscle wastage will occur. At such high intensities, even after eating a big bowl of porridge, this could occur within as short a duration as 30 minutes, other factors dependent.

The consensus of opinion, whether CT or HIIT, is to eat something immediately following your workout – Just like you would also do if you were engaging in a strength training programme.

Anaerobic training, such as HIIT, depletes glycogen stores. These stores need replacing as quickly as possible. Food rich in carbohydrate and protein should be taken as a matter of priority. This will ensure that fat burning through EPOC is maximised, while lean muscle tissue is preserved.

I really don't want to make things any more complicated than they need to be when the fact is that it's all quite simple.

I'll also make a quick point on hydration - It's best to arrive for your HIIT workouts fully hydrated. This will ensure you're in a good state for training. Recovery periods are also ideal for taking in yet more water. And of course, any lost water should be replaced at the conclusion of the HIIT workout. Regular sips are far more preferential to infrequent gulps.

HIIT Pitfalls

As with any form of exercise, injuries are always possible. The best advice is always to take the necessary precautions in order to avoid an injury. Make sure you use suitable footwear which is comfortable. More importantly, as I've already described, please ensure you carry out all necessary warm ups, cool downs and post workout stretches. Of course accidents can always happen, in which case there's not a lot you can legislate for. But you can certainly safeguard yourself against what you can control which are injuries relating to poor exercise preparation.

It's perhaps unfair to compare injury rates between HIIT and CT participants owing to the greater time CT participants exercise and therefore allowing for more opportunities for tripping up, falling or straining etc. In fact, I have not been able to find any studies that directly compare the two groups specifically when it comes to injuries. I did however come across a study that compared injury rates between recreational Swedish sprinters, middle distance runners and long distance/marathon runners [19].

A total of 60 runners from all groups were followed and monitored for a year. Of these runners, a total of 55 injuries were reported between 39 runners. Per 1000 hours of training – The injury rate was 2.5 for the long distance/marathon runners and 5.6 for both the middle distance runners and sprinters.

We can see here that the chance of being injured during a HIIT sprinting session is still quite remote, yet unfortunately more than double the likelihood suffered from marathon runners. I will add that if you're reading this book, you are less likely to be a keen marathon runner due to extreme endurance activities being at the opposite end of the fitness spectrum.

I will also add that during the study, 72% of injuries from all groups were sustained due to a training error. Unfortunately, these are the things you just can't plan for other than ensuring you're wearing robust footwear and remaining vigilant whilst training.

What were the most common preventable injuries? Foot sores were the most problematic for the marathon runners and backache and hip problems for the middle distance runners. The sprinters suffered most from hamstring strains which is understandable considering the explosive nature of sprinting. Secondly, they suffered from tendinitis of the Achilles tendon. We will cover both these most common sprinting related injuries now.

Of course, this may not even be relevant to you depending on which mode of HIIT you choose to dedicate the majority of your time to. Though as you know, I am extremely biased toward sprinting myself and I will also make the assumption that most readers of this book will also be heavily inclined toward sprinting for their HIIT fix. I have also stated earlier that switching training modes is beneficial for all HIIT advocates. But I will also add that any type of jumping as well as many of the kettlebell exercises also involve comparable forms of explosive activity and thus place the hamstrings under similar potential risk from strains.

Hamstring Strains

In most cases, hamstring strains are preventable. The best way to avoid them is by warming up thoroughly before you begin the high intensity segments of your HIIT workouts (we have already discussed the other benefits of proper warm ups). You should also thoroughly stretch all major muscle groups following your workouts, which should include a period of developmental stretching for the hamstrings (as already discussed).

Another common cause of hamstring strains is a hamstrings/quadriceps muscle imbalance. Everybody has weaker hamstrings than quadriceps but potential problems may arrive when the hamstrings/quadriceps strength ratio reaches 60:100, when the hamstrings are only 60% or below the strength of the quadriceps. Though please take note that ideally our imbalance should better reflect 75:100. This imbalance may well be a problem for us because the straightening of the knee joint (carried out by the quadriceps) may be too forceful and so the hamstrings, which act as antagonists and stabilise the knee joint could be damaged during the process of the many explosive contractions we perform during HIIT.

If you're worried, then discovering the degree of your imbalance (everybody has one) is easy. If you have access to a gym then simply ascertain your 1 rep maximum on both the leg extension and leg curl machines which utilise your quadriceps and hamstrings respectively. If you're only able to curl (hamstrings) 60 percent or less than what you can extend (quadriceps) then I highly suggest you undertake strength training exercises targeting your hamstrings. I also suggest you carry out this test using both legs together as well as each leg individually. Strength will most likely differ between legs and one is more likely to injure the weaker hamstring than the stronger one.

Ensuring your hamstrings/quadriceps muscle imbalance is within an acceptable range will also help with flexibility, range of motion of the knee joint and also protect your knees from other potential problems. Indeed studies [20] have found that subjects undergoing anterior cruciate ligament reconstruction were more likely to have hamstrings/quadriceps muscle imbalances than control groups. This imbalance most likely represented a compromised ability of the hamstrings to stabilise the knee joint through the full range of motion.

Of course there are many other possible injuries you could sustain while sprinting or using one of the other HIIT modes, though covering all of those would be impossible. However, by undertaking the correct starting procedures as described and by ascertaining the nature of your imbalance (and then taking action if necessary) then you are safeguarding yourself as much as possible against future hamstring and knee problems.

Achilles Tendinitis

You can actually get tendinitis in a range of areas where there is excessive repetitive movement such as the major joints. Tendons can become inflamed and gradually tighten until fibres begin to tear. For HIIT participants, tendinitis is most likely to occur in the Achilles tendon, and this is not necessarily specific only to sprinters as most HIIT modes, and not just HIIT but CT also, involve rhythmic and repetitive movements.

Although it's not completely understood why tendinitis occurs, it is thought that overuse is perhaps the main contributing factor and it accounts for around 15% of running injuries. Almost all the force generated when you "toe off" the ground during running/sprinting is transmitted by the Achilles tendon. Naturally, the faster you run, the more force and therefore strain you are putting on the Achilles.

Symptoms include a weakness at the joint, swelling and redness. Of course pain is also a symptom and thus will render you unable to train for anywhere between a few days to several weeks.

Naturally, if you feel you have tendinitis then you should pay a visit to your doctor as soon as possible in order to prevent it from becoming even more severe. As always though, prevention is better than cure and you can safeguard yourself as much as possible from Achilles tendinitis by:

- Warming up thoroughly.
- Recognising the differences between an ache caused by lactic acid and an ache caused by an injury (not always easy).
- Wearing comfortable footwear.
- Ensuring good technique.
- Warming down.
- Post workout stretching – This is the most important preventative measure as stretching will lengthen the tendon connection. This will lessen the pulling on the tendon attachment to the bone.

It's only right that I include information about possible injuries resulting from HIIT for reasons of thoroughness. You should be aware of the potential pitfalls as well as the benefits. Having said that, and as we can see from the above study [19], the chances of sustaining an injury during a HIIT session or as a result of many HIIT sessions is still very remote.

Sample HIIT Workouts

Now comes the fun part. It's time to get out there and start doing some HIIT.

The next few pages demonstrate a small number of hypothetical protocols, which may be used when running outside. They are merely to demonstrate some of the many possibilities for variance. You should get out there and have fun designing your very own HIIT route.

Of course everybody's track, route or protocol will be different. There are many variables that will depend on what your chosen route will look like such as your locale, skill level and HIIT protocol.

Sample HIIT Track 1

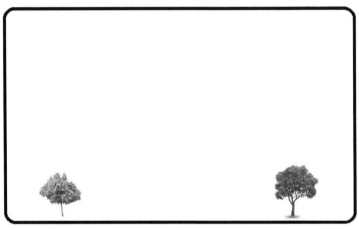

1, 3, 5, 7 etc   2, 4, 6, 8 etc

I would first take a primary lap to warm up; utilising a fast walk and then going into a comfortable jog.

1. When you hit the tree, you know what to do. Give it all you've got.
2. When you hit tree 2, walk. But keep the walk brisk. This should last anywhere between 2 – 4 minutes.
3. You're back at the first tree again - Sprint.
4. Etc...

Sample HIIT Track 2

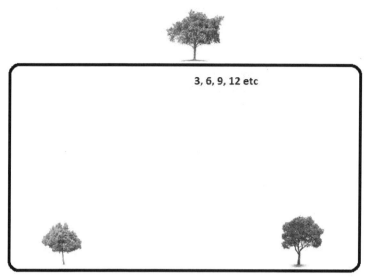

3, 6, 9, 12 etc

1, 4, 7, 10 etc   **2, 5, 8, 11 etc**

In track 2 we're adding a bit of variety. After our walk periods, we're going to take things into a gentle jog prior to the all-out sprint interval.

Remember your primary warm up lap, walking and jogging.

1. Sprint
2. Walk
3. Jog
4. Sprint
5. Walk
6. Jog etc

Sample HIIT Track 3

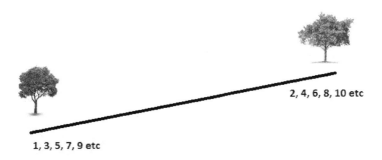

2, 4, 6, 8, 10 etc

1, 3, 5, 7, 9 etc

This track is more advanced. Sprinting uphill is what you should eventually be aiming to do as there are very few better or faster ways of achieving a maximal heart rate level than this.

If you walk straight back down after arriving at the top, often the recovery period will have been extremely short. Feel free to walk back to the start position in an arc to give yourself a little more recovery time.

This is very intense. After you've finished your final uphill sprint, don't forget to have a gradual cool down involving a short jog and a walk prior to a post workout stretch.

Sample HIIT Track 4

Moving away from the local park and onto the road:

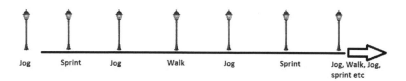

This time we're using lamp posts as our markers and this time we have a different pattern of intervals as you can see.

Of course, as I hope I've explained. You really don't need to follow these examples. Feel free to create whatever course you desire.

You could even ignore the lamp posts or the trees entirely and do your HIIT according to how you feel at the time; Fartlek protocol.

As long as you're elevating your heart rate as high as possible and you're giving it your all then you can't really go wrong with HIIT. Listen to your body and go with what it's telling you.

Obviously, if you own a bike then the above *track 4* will also be perfect for cycling.

Sample HIIT Protocol 5

The following HIIT protocols have been tried and tested by myself and my clients over the years. All the following protocols are ideal for any of the HIIT modes.

High Intensity (seconds)	Rest (seconds)
10	50
10	50
10	50

High Intensity (seconds)	Rest (seconds)
15	45
15	45
15	45

High Intensity (seconds)	Rest (seconds)
20	40
20	40
20	40

High Intensity (seconds)	Rest (seconds)
25	35
25	35
25	35

High Intensity (seconds)	Rest (seconds)
30	30
30	30
30	30

Easy

Hardest

Each of these designs is fairly rigid. If you're starting out then you should begin at the top and work your way down as you become fitter and more experienced.

You'll notice that each line of text represents 1 minute. Each minute is made up of a high intensity period and a rest period. I've included only the first three minutes of each session. But obviously you would carry out anywhere between 20 – 30 minutes of activity.

Why not start at the top for session one; carrying out 10 seconds of high intensity work followed by 50 seconds of rest.

For your first session you could carry out 20 minutes of exercise. For your second session - 25 minutes and for the final session - 30 minutes.

Then for the next time you try this protocol you could begin with the second box down; 15 seconds of high intensity work and 45 seconds of rest. However, you could return to 20 minutes of activity in total and build it back up to 30 minutes over the course of the next few sessions.

If you carry on with this pattern, you are constantly testing yourself, things are becoming slightly more intensive with each training session and everything remains truly interesting.

Completing the programme should take a total of 15 HIIT workouts, by which time you'll have really noticed the difference in your abilities.

If you're able to carry out the dreaded 30:30 splits then you have my congratulations.

Sample HIIT Protocol 6

The protocol below is easy to understand. It follows a simple pattern of 30 seconds high intensity followed by 1 minute of rest.

This 1:2 ratio of hard work to rest is actually an intermediate to advanced level so it's something to build up to.

Don't feel you need to stop at 19.5 minutes, but feel free to build up to 30 minutes over time.

Of course, this protocol can be used with any HIIT mode.

High Intensity	Recovery
0:00 - 0:30	0:31 - 1:30
1:31 - 2:00	02:01 - 03:00
03:01 - 03:30	03:31 - 04:30
04:31 - 05:00	05:01 - 06:00
06:01 - 06:30	06:31 - 07:30
07:31 - 08:00	08:01 - 09:00
09:01 - 09:30	09:31 - 10:30
10:31 - 11:00	11:01 - 12:00
12:01 - 12:30	12:31 - 13:30
13:31 - 14:00	14:01 - 15:00
15:01 - 15:30	15:31 - 16:30
16:31 - 17:00	17:01 - 18:00
18:01 - 18:30	18:31 - 19:30

Sample HIIT Protocol 7

High Intensity (seconds)	Recovery (seconds)
10	50
10	50
15	45
15	45
20	40
20	40
25	35
25	35
30	30
30	30
35	25
35	25
40	20
40	20
45	15
45	15
50	10
50	10

Total Time = 18 minutes

This is where things get really interesting. This protocol becomes gradually more advanced as the HIIT session progresses.

Each line represents one minute. Every two minutes the ratio of high intensity work increases as the rest period decreases.

As you approach the end of the protocol, things clearly become incredibly difficult, even for highly advanced participants.

So why not set yourself a challenge?

When you progress to *Sample HIIT Protocol 7*, I would suggest trying to make it further through the protocol on each subsequent session. Very few people can make it through a workout such as this, but it can be fun trying make it through an extra 10 – 20 seconds on each subsequent session. Just remember to record your progress.

Feel that burn.

Common HIIT Questions

Question: I've tried HIIT a couple of times and on both occasions I've had a headache following the session. What am I doing wrong?

From speaking to clients and friends, I believe that HIIT induced headaches are more common for those just starting out than for those who've been partaking for a while. Common sense would have that the headaches are due to adjusting to the sudden change in intensity. Consider taking longer recovery periods between high intensity intervals in order to more gradually ease your body (and head) into the new regime.

Though let's make no mistake – They are rare.

You should be able to bear the headaches out and within a few sessions they should abate in the vast majority of cases. If they continue then as always a doctor should be consulted.

It would be unfair to say that headaches are limited to just HIIT because they are not. A simple online search for "exercise induced headaches" should prove this.

A preventive approach should be considered and as always, there is nothing special to preventive actions – Just plain common sense.

Ensure you're hydrated before doing any physical activity and remain hydrated throughout your workouts. Recovery periods are ideal opportunities to take a quick gulp of water.

Top up your glycogen levels with a light snack before your workout and reread the section on *HIIT Nutrition.* It seems common that those who suffer from exercise induced headaches are low on blood sugar during their workouts. We need glycogen for HIIT. It's our fuel.

Finally I would enquire as to the nature of your job and does it involve frequent periods hunched over a computer or desk. Desk bound jobs can over the years result in a tightening of the upper back and neck muscles. Tight muscles in these areas can cause headaches. The remedy is one I think you'll enjoy. Book yourself in to see a sports massage therapist and have the area ironed out.

Question: Could you clarify the difference between interval training and HIIT?

Interval training can refer to any form of training where the intensities are altered, usually between high intensities and recovery periods. Interval training *can,* but not necessarily encompass *high intensity interval training.* In general when people say *interval training,* they are referring to high intensity periods of between 75 – 90% of maximal heart rate. When people talk about HIIT, they are referring to 95%+. But for the purpose of this book – And for when *I* talk about HIIT – I'm referring to *all-out.* I'm talking about 100% balls to the wall, can't do anymore even if you paid me kind of intensity.

Question: I've been inactive for several years – Is it safe to jump straight into a HIIT regime?

While the human body can adapt positively in a short period of time, given extreme enough stimuli, it can also degenerate shockingly quickly if we remain inactive. Have you ever watched astronauts on the space station on TV? They spend up to two hours, six days a week on cycle ergometers, strapped to treadmills and carrying out heavy weights routines with specially built machines in order to prevent their muscles from withering away. Then when they return to earth, they undergo long periods of rehabilitation in order to rebuild the muscle mass they lost due to their being little to no load bearing on their bones for many months. In fact NASA themselves have been experimenting with HIIT in order to get the most results from the least time when in space. They admit that the bulk of the two hours spent exercising daily is in fact carried out strength training. Looks like HIIT has the NASA stamp of approval.

The point is that degeneration or muscle wastage can occur quickly – Perhaps in as short a time period as 3 weeks, other variables depending, and of course you don't need to be in space to feel these negative effects.

The good news is that if you've had a reasonable level of past fitness, then getting back to your old fitness levels, or a stage where you can safely carry out HIIT sessions will take less time than if you were starting out having never been in reasonable shape. I'm sure you've heard of muscle memory? This is what it's referring to.

However, a common sense approach should be taken when easing yourself back into a HIIT regime. I would recommend first carrying out a CT workout or two and be your own judge as to how you feel – Listen to your body. If you're able to jog at a reasonable pace for 30 minutes, then in my opinion you're fine to start sprinting at 100% balls-to-the-wall once again.

In this book I've referenced studies where cardiac patients have been used as subjects. Unless there's something exceptional holding you back, then the vast majority of people will not have problems with a few brief high intensity intervals. Remember that you're in full control of your interval periods. Simply expand the duration of your recovery periods and judge each interval as it comes. Listen to your body.

Question: Are apps recommended for HIIT workouts?

Yes, especially if you're skipping or using kettlebells or bodyweight circuits. There are many apps available, but they all do the same basic thing, which is to act as a timer. Simply input the length of the high intensity periods as well as your recovery periods and set it to 'go' and it will chime as directed. Some apps will even allow you to listen to music as you exercise and will chime over the song.

Question: I'm pregnant – Can I still do HIIT?

Well this depends entirely on you. Everybody is different. You should however pay extremely close attention to the advice given by your doctor as they will take your individual situation into consideration.

What I do know for a fact is that running is ok during pregnancy but that it's fairly common for painful sensations to be felt approaching the mid-stages. This demonstrates why it's hard to give a definitive answer as every woman will be different.

Bottom line – Listen to your body. If you feel able to carry out HIIT – especially during the early stages, then there'll be no problems. If you already do HIIT regularly then you'll be even less likely to have problems due to your pregnancy.

You may though like to consider a slightly lower intensity protocol and with an exercise mode, such as walking or swimming, especially once you enter the mid stages of pregnancy.

Question: I'm no longer a young man. Is there any more advice you can give for seniors wanting to begin a HIIT routine for the first time?

Again, this depends on the individual. If you already have a good cardiovascular fitness base then switching to HIIT will be much easier. If this is indeed the case then I recommend beginning with a less intense HIIT protocol such as the Little Method or even an interval training protocol with only two or three bursts of high intensity at around 85% of your maximal heart rate. Take your time with recovery periods and only increase the intensity again when ready. It's very important to listen to your body. Begin with a low impact HIIT mode such as swimming or walking.

If you're beginning from a low fitness base then I would suggest first partaking in a few CT workouts. You should aim to keep your heart rate at around 70% of its maximum. But there's no need to put off using an interval training protocol for long. When it's all said and done – You'll achieve much more from HIIT than from CT so there's no point in stalling. Begin by using between two and four high intensity intervals at a maximal heart rate of between 80 – 90%. Utilise longer recovery periods. With each subsequent session either increase the intensity of the high intensity periods, decrease the duration of recovery periods or add extra intervals.

The above advice can actually apply to a range of "at risk" people who are nervous about the thought of exercising at high intensities. Let me reassure you that high intensity exercise is extremely safe. It's far better to undertake high intensity exercise under controlled conditions, where you're prepared for it having warmed up, than having to suddenly exert yourself in an unprepared state because of an unforeseen circumstance or an emergency.

Question: Are there any other benefits to HIIT that you're holding back from us?

Well yes there are and this would be a good place to mention them. HIIT is becoming more and more popular every day and with that comes new research from universities all over the world. As a HIIT enthusiast, I like to keep my eye on this new research.

Some recent studies have been comparing HIIT with CT on the effects of blood pressure, heart disease, diabetes, strokes as well as other conditions. Although this research is in its infancy, you won't be surprised to learn that HIIT is winning out against CT.

Given that HIIT yields greater improvements over CT for increases in VO2 max, one can see how this would be helpful for those suffering from cardiovascular disease, or heart disease. Considering that heart disease is the number 1 cause of death in America, the potential here is huge.

Preliminary research is also showing that vigorous exercise is helping to reduce stroke risk in men and women and is also helping stroke victims recover faster. However, moderate and even moderate to heavy exercise has not been found to have a protective effect. Did you ever imagine that HIIT could even help reduce the risk from strokes, when CT does not? The future for HIIT research is extremely exciting indeed.

Going all the way back to the beginning of this book, when we spoke about evolution, one should never be surprised to learn that what is natural for us as human beings, will protect us in life. This is how nature intended us to be. Short bursts of high intensity exercise is far more natural than jogging at a medium pace for hours on end.

It is my belief that HIIT will also improve an individual's motor skills (balance, coordination, reaction time, power, agility) over and above what CT will do. This will be especially true if the individual engages in a range of HIIT modes with kettlebell and bodyweight circuits being amongst the best for this. This is because the individual will be relying on balance and skill for many of those exercises such as kettlebell swings, squat jumps, box jumps, lunge jumps etc. Having improved motor skills will benefit individuals long into their later years. One study [21] has shown that poor explosive power in the legs was a future predictor of falling frequency in elderly women.

Clearly there are many more areas where research needs to take place and I expect this research to come to fruition as HIIT becomes ever more popular.

Conclusion

I'm glad you've made it this far and now comes the fun part.

Get out into your local gym or park and HIIT it up. Results are sure to come far quicker and far easier (ok, maybe not easier) than by using any other training method in existence.

It's a scandal that too few people know about, or ever participate in HIIT. A casual observance of exercisers in the local gym or joggers on the street should confirm this to you.

Hopefully things will change, that's down to us to spread the word.

If you've enjoyed this book and feel that others would benefit from the knowledge within then please feel free to leave an honest review on the sales page where you purchased it.

Whatever your goals for HIIT are, I hope you achieve them and I wish you all the success in health and fitness.

References

[1]   http://www.ncbi.nlm.nih.gov/pubmed/11070099

Albert CM. et al. (2000). Triggering of sudden death from cardiac causes by vigorous exertion. *The New England Journal of Medicine*. 343(19):1355-61.

[2]   http://www.ncbi.nlm.nih.gov/pubmed/21360405

Bartlett JD. et al. (2011). High-intensity interval running is perceived to be more enjoyable than moderate-intensity continuous exercise: implications for exercise adherence. *Journal of Sports Sciences*. 29(6):547-53.

[3]   http://www.ncbi.nlm.nih.gov/pubmed/20473222

Macpherson RE. et al. (2011). Run sprint interval training improves aerobic performance but not maximal cardiac output. *Medicine and Science in Sports and Exercise*. 43(1):115-22.

[4]   http://www.ncbi.nlm.nih.gov/pubmed/2305702

Tremblay A. et al. (1990). Effect of intensity of physical activity on body fatness and fat distribution. *The American Journal of Clinical Nutrition*. 51(2):153-7.

[5]   http://www.ncbi.nlm.nih.gov/pubmed/17001221

Wisloff U. et al. (2006). A single weekly bout of exercise may reduce cardiovascular mortality: how little pain for cardiac gain? 'The HUNT study, Norway'. *European Journal of Cardiovascular Prevention and Rehabilitation.* 13(5):798-804

[6]   http://www.ncbi.nlm.nih.gov/pubmed/19088769

Perry CG. et al. (2008). High-intensity aerobic interval training increases fat and carbohydrate metabolic capacities in human skeletal muscle. *Applied Physiology, Nutrition and Metabolism.* 33(6):1112-23.

[7]   http://www.ncbi.nlm.nih.gov/pubmed/17170203

Talanian JL. et al. (1985). Two weeks of high-intensity aerobic interval training increases the capacity for fat oxidation during exercise in women. *Journal of Applied Physiology.* 102(4):1439-47.

[8]   http://www.ncbi.nlm.nih.gov/pubmed/16825308

Gibala MJ. et al. (2006). Short-term sprint interval versus traditional endurance training: similar initial adaptations in human skeletal muscle and exercise performance. *The Journal of Physiology.* 575(3):901-11.

[9]   http://etd-submit.etsu.edu/etd/theses/available/etd-0412101-214442/unrestricted/king0417.pdf

King JW. et al. (2001). A Comparison of the Effects of Interval Training vs. Continuous Training on Weight Loss and Body Composition in Obese Pre-Menopausal Women. A thesis presented to the faculty of the Department of

Physical Education, Exercise, and Sports Sciences East Tennessee State University.

[10]   http://www.ncbi.nlm.nih.gov/pubmed/8028502

Tremblay A. et al. (1994). Impact of exercise intensity on body fatness and skeletal muscle metabolism. *Metabolism: Clinical and Experimental*. 43(7):814-8.

[11]
        http://blog.sme.sk/blog/3928/155928/Warburton_ CAD.pdf

Darren ER. et al. (2005). Effectiveness of High-Intensity Interval Training for the Rehabilitation of Patients With Coronary Artery Disease. *American Journal of Cardiology*. 95:1080-1084.

[12]   http://www.ncbi.nlm.nih.gov/pubmed/8897392

Tabata I. et al. (1996). Effects of moderate-intensity endurance and high-intensity intermittent training on anaerobic capacity and VO2max. *Medicine and Science in Sports and Exercise*. 28(10):1327-30.

[13]   http://www.ncbi.nlm.nih.gov/pubmed/1553453

Schwarz L. et al. (1992). Changes in beta-endorphin levels in response to aerobic and anaerobic exercise. *Sports Medicine*. 13(1):25-36.

[14]   http://www.ncbi.nlm.nih.gov/pubmed/17548726

Wisloff U. (2007). Superior cardiovascular effect of aerobic interval training versus moderate continuous training in heart failure patients: a randomized study. *Circulation.* 115(24):3086-94.

[15]   http://www.ncbi.nlm.nih.gov/pubmed/16237625

McManus AM. et al. (2005). Improving aerobic power in primary school boys: a comparison of continuous and interval training. *International Journal of Sports Medicine.* 26(9):781-6.

[16]   http://www.ncbi.nlm.nih.gov/pubmed/16469933

Burgomaster KA. (2006). Effect of short-term sprint interval training on human skeletal muscle carbohydrate metabolism during exercise and time-trial performance. *Journal of Applied Physiology.* 100(6):2041-7.

[17]   http://www.ncbi.nlm.nih.gov/pubmed/10331896

Stepto NK. et al. (1999). Effects of different interval-training programs on cycling time-trial performance. *Medicine and Science in Sports and Exercise.* 31(5):736-41.

[18]
    http://jp.physoc.org/content/early/2010/01/20/jp
hysiol.2009.181743

Little JP. et al. (2010). A practical model of low-volume high-intensity interval training induces mitochondrial biogenesis in human skeletal muscle: potential mechanisms. *The Journal of Physiology.* 10.1113/jphysiol.2009.181743.

[19] http://ajs.sagepub.com/content/15/2/168

Lysholm J. et al. (1987). Injuries in runners. *American Journal of Sports Medicine.* 15(2):168-171.

[20] http://www.ncbi.nlm.nih.gov/pubmed/15377966

Hiemstra LA. et al. (2004). Hamstring and quadriceps strength balance in normal and hamstring anterior cruciate ligament-reconstructed subjects. *Clinical Journal of Sport Medicine: Official Journal of the Canadian Academy of Sport Medicine.* 14(5):274-80.

[21] http://www.ncbi.nlm.nih.gov/pubmed/11937474

Skelton DA. et al. (2002). Explosive power and asymmetry in leg muscle function in frequent fallers and non-fallers aged over 65. *Age and Ageing.* 31(2):119-25.

Also By James Driver

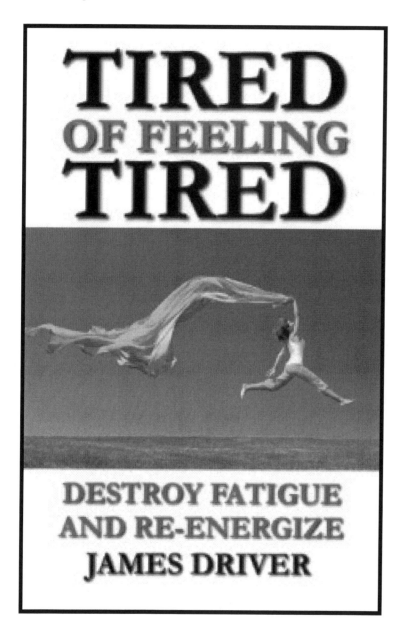

TIRED
OF FEELING
TIRED

**DESTROY FATIGUE
AND RE-ENERGIZE
JAMES DRIVER**

Feeling tired, lethargic or fatigued is one of the main reasons we visit the doctor. However, we are often told there's nothing wrong with us.

Chronic fatigue is the feeling of being low on energy at various points during the day for no reason whatsoever. Is this something you feel on a regular basis?

Do you struggle to pull yourself out of bed in the morning?
Do you find sleeping at night difficult?
Do you find yourself taking frequent midday naps?
Are you depressed due to your feelings of fatigue?
Are you stressed out because of this?
Are your days not as productive as they could be?
Do you pass up invitations to go out with friends due to feeling tired and fatigued?

If so then it's likely you suffer from chronic fatigue or some other condition that causes you to feel low on energy.

In this book you will discover:

What condition, if any you may have.
If not, then how to pin-point your lifestyle habits that are making you feel fatigued.
Exactly what you can do to give yourself more energy than you've ever had before.

The author James Driver believes in making positive lifestyle changes that are all natural, healthy and drug free.

This is the way towards an all-round, healthy life with an abundance of energy.

Tired of Feeling Tired is not full of medical language that is hard to understand and neither is it overly lengthy but is straight to the point. Tired of Feeling Tired is not for the PhD student but is instead for the individual who is suffering from this invisible condition.

See also a case study of a professional dancer who suffered from fatigue for many years and how she overcame it.

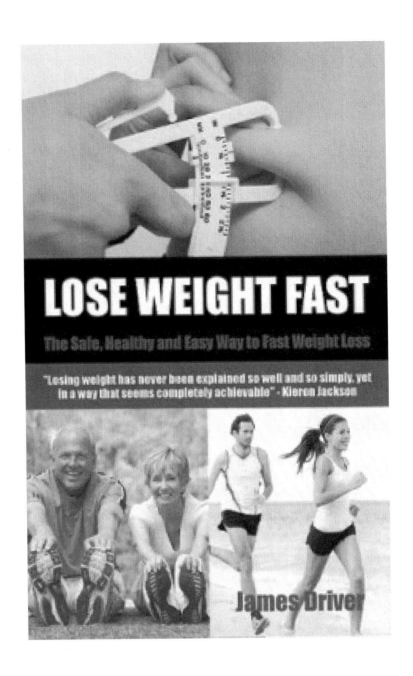

LOSE WEIGHT FAST

The Safe, Healthy and Easy Way to Fast Weight Loss

"Losing weight has never been explained so well and so simply, yet in a way that seems completely achievable" - Kieron Jackson

James Driver

Most methods that aim to help you lose weight fast just aren't very healthy. They all seem to take a "too much – too soon" approach which instead guarantees long term failure for anybody who wants a healthy weight loss plan.

There are indeed methods that can help you succeed at fast weight loss which also remain safe, effective and healthy. These weight loss or more to the point...fat loss methods are always the best methods.

In Lose Weight Fast, you will learn an overall approach to healthy fat loss, taking into account your overall diet and eating patterns. Then you will learn the one exercise technique that the author James Driver, a personal trainer of 12 years knows to be the single most effective method of burning fat from your body.

Together, these two shifts in your lifestyle will have the rapid effect of melting the fat straight from your body and in a period of time you never thought possible.

18611516R00133

Made in the USA
Middletown, DE
13 March 2015